DIAGNOSTIC BRONCHOSCOPY

For Churchill Livingstone

Publisher   Michael Parkinson
Editor   Jane Starling
Production Controller   Mrs Lesley W. Small
Designer   Design Resources Unit
Sales Promotion Executive   Marion Pollock

DIAGNOSTIC BRONCHOSCOPY

A TEACHING MANUAL

PETER STRADLING
M.D.(Lond.), F.R.C.P., F.R.P.S.

Lately Director of the Chest Clinic and Senior Lecturer
in Respiratory Diseases: Royal Postgraduate Medical
School, Hammersmith Hospital, London, UK

SIXTH EDITION

With the assistance of

JOHN R STRADLING
B.Sc., M.D.(Lond.), F.R.C.P.

Wellcome Senior Research Fellow
and Consultant Physician,
Chest Unit, Churchill Hospital,
Oxford, UK

CHURCHILL LIVINGSTONE
EDINBURGH LONDON MELBOURNE NEW YORK AND TOKYO 1991

CHURCHILL LIVINGSTONE
Medical Division of Longman Group UK Limited

Distributed in the United States of America by
Churchill Livingstone Inc., 650 Avenue of the Americas,
New York, N.Y. 10011, and by associated companies, branches
and representatives throughout the world.

First edition 1968
Second edition 1973
Third edition 1976
Fourth edition 1981
Fifth edition 1986
Sixth edition 1991
   Reprinted 1993

ISBN 0-443-04293-4

The
publisher's
policy is to use
paper manufactured
from sustainable forests

Printed in Hong Kong
CPL/02

'More is missed by not looking than by not knowing'

THOMAS MCCRAE
1870–1935

ACKNOWLEDGEMENTS

With any project there are usually many people who, directly or indirectly, contribute to its successful conclusion. To all those who have helped, in whatever sphere and however indirectly, to produce six editions of this book, I am truly grateful, and regret the impossibility of mentioning them all by name.

Some have contributed so importantly, however, that I take especial pleasure in acknowledging my deep indebtedness to them, and first I must put the late Robert Laird FRCS, and the late John Jackson FRCS, surgeons who, painstakingly and with great forbearance, introduced a physician to the art of bronchoscopy. Subsequently, the cheerful, willing and skilful co-operation of the Anaesthetic and Operating Theatre Staffs made my bronchoscopy sessions a weekly pleasure. The Ward Staffs also played a big part in making the procedure acceptable to the patients. Many of these patients were referred from other clinicians, particularly Drs Graham Poole, Alexander Ferguson and Graham Richardson, to whom I am extremely grateful.

A major contribution to the book is the series of line drawings. These are largely the excellent work of the late Miss Sylvia Treadgold AIMBI, to whom I am deeply indebted. I am very grateful to Miss Jo Dyer B.A. (Hons), MMAA, for additional drawings in this edition.

Any inaccuracies in the text of this edition remain entirely my responsibility, but they have certainly been reduced by the invaluable constructive criticism of the manuscript by my son John. He has also taken a major part in revising the chapter on fibreoptic bronchoscopy. I am very grateful to him for the time and attention so willingly given.

Although publishing is a publisher's duty, this should not be taken for granted and it is with pleasure that I record the patience, meticulous attention to detail and courtesy of the staff of Churchill Livingstone.

Finally, I wish to record my deepest gratitude to my wife for bearing with me during the months that this edition has been in preparation, for constructive criticism and for help with proof reading.

CONTENTS

CHAPTER 1

INTRODUCTION

No physician specialising in respiratory medicine today is considered adequately trained unless competent with the bronchoscope: the problem is learning the art.

While nothing can replace personal clinical practice and experience, access to a representative collection of illustrations helps to solve the problem. Normal anatomy and a variety of pathological conditions can be studied in a few hours to give preparatory knowledge, albeit superficial, which would take months to obtain in any other way. Rescrutiny of illustrations, after lesions have been seen in reality, further helps to consolidate knowledge and experience. The colour photographs reproduced in this book, forming a representative collection of normal and common abnormal findings, were all taken during routine bronchoscopy sessions and have been selected with the learner's needs in view.

It should be stressed that the aim of the work is strictly limited. Technique is discussed only in outline on the assumption that a practical apprenticeship will be served. No attempt is made to produce an exhaustive atlas, to review literature, to deal with the special problems of bronchoscopy in children, to discuss the complicated subject of foreign body removal, or to advise on available apparatus. Such matters are either dealt with in other publications, or will depend on the personal preference of the operator and his teacher.

This book is produced to help the student of bronchoscopy appreciate the true value of the investigation and learn his way about the normal and abnormal bronchial tree; it is not an advanced textbook.

Today, most respiratory physicians are competent with the fibrescope but very few young bronchoscopists have experience with the rigid bronchoscope. This is considered less than ideal, for the instruments have complementary advantages and limitations which require competence with both. Thus a chapter on rigid tube bronchoscopy is retained.

However, variations in bronchoscopic technique do not affect the value of this pictorial monograph: the findings are the same, however viewed. In this connection, the learner is advised constantly to think of the bronchial tree as a three-dimensional entity; *not* in terms of two-dimensional pictures. Not only will this assist in handling the instruments, but will greatly reduce problems of orientation if changing the technique of operating, or viewing photographs taken with patients postured differently from that to which he is accustomed.

No photographs taken through the bronchofibrescope have been included because the limitations imposed by fibre bundle image transmission make them markedly inferior to those obtained by the best rigid optics. Furthermore, pathological states occurring in small bronchi, only visible through the fibre-scope, are no different, except in size, from those illustrated here. Photographs of the more peripheral normal anatomy are also considered unnecessary. The details are so varied and yet the general plan so comparable, whichever segment is studied, that the large number of similar photographs needed would be confusing and of little clinical value.

The text has been kept short and dogmatic to serve as an introduction to each group of photographs, which are then individually and briefly discussed. Although taken through a rigid bronchoscope with the patient supine, they have, for this edition, been inverted because it is appreciated that the majority of bronchoscopies are now performed with the operator facing his patient. An exception is made in Chapter 4 when discussing the introduction of the rigid bronchoscope. Annotated drawings are provided which serve to locate the items of major interest in each photograph. To help in appreciating the anatomy, perspective and spatial relationships, small conventional plans of the bronchial tree have been added. An arrow indicates the position of the telescope objective lens, and the direction in which it was pointing, when the photograph was taken. No attempt has been made to draw intraluminal lesions on these plans, but when the anatomy differs from the prevailing pattern, or has been distorted, this has been indicated where possible: distortions in the sagittal plane, however, cannot be expressed in this way (for example Plates 97, 98 & 102).

Approximately a fifth of the photographic plates are deliberately devoted to normality because this has a wide range and is very often as difficult for the beginner to appreciate as are the varieties of pathology: furthermore, patients with healthy mucosa are rarely bronchoscoped and thus the opportunity to see the normal occurs infrequently. Among the pathological conditions, pride of place is given to those arising most commonly; inflammatory changes, bronchial distortions and the manifestations of bronchial carcinoma. It is more important that the learner should thoroughly understand normality, and the *common* pathological conditions, than become confused by rarities. A few unusual conditions are included to whet the appetite.

CHAPTER 2

INDICATIONS FOR BRONCHOSCOPY

Bronchoscopy is probably an underused procedure, usually because its diagnostic potential is underrated. In some appropriate instances the investigation is not thought of and therefore not undertaken. In others the supposed danger and discomfort are greatly exaggerated. Long discussions may take place on the advisability of bronchoscopy, so wasting much time and effort. In fact, contra-indications are few. Modern techniques of anaesthesia, either local or general, and of ventilation make the procedure so safe that a patient must be gravely ill, or have quite gross reduction in respiratory reserve, before bronchoscopy becomes dangerous. Clearly, in the immediately hopeless case, investigations would be inhuman; a similar argument applies to great age and frailty. Certain patients, with advanced superior vena caval obstruction, and therefore urgently needing radiotherapy, should have their bronchoscopy delayed until after treatment has started and there has been some subsidence of neck swelling: bronchoscopy before radiation can sometimes lead to trouble from postoperative laryngeal oedema, or excessive bleeding when a biopsy is attempted.

Bronchoscopy, a safe and invaluable investigation, should be performed very readily. If this policy is followed many unsuspected diagnoses will be made, suspected diagnoses confirmed, much time saved and distress often avoided. To illustrate this wide scope of bronchoscopy is the aim of the following discussion of indications.

The patient's history

The patient's present symptom, or symptoms, together with the story of the illness, are of paramount diagnostic importance and must be listened to with the utmost care. *The clinician should be prepared to undertake bronchoscopy on the history alone.* It is not sufficiently well known that gross pathology (for example tumour or radiolucent foreign body) can be present in a large airway without producing any physical signs or radiological change (Plates 145, 150, 153, 174 & 217). Nevertheless the discerning physician will often be suspicious on first hearing the patient's story. One suggestive symptom alone should lead to action, but multiple symptoms strengthen the indication for bronchoscopy. In particular, so much information may be obtained bronchoscopically in cases of bronchial carcinoma that this examination should be carried out in all patients where there is the slightest suspicion of the disease, particularly if they are, or have been, heavy smokers.

Individual symptoms are discussed further in the following sections.

Haemoptysis

This is a major and frequent indication but careful history taking and examination will exclude a proportion of patients from further consideration because the bleeding is clearly not of bronchial origin. A further group will have presented with a very small single bleed, presumed pulmonary, normal postero-anterior and lateral radiographs, no history of smoking and perhaps a recent simple infection: to bronchoscope all such patients routinely (arguably the ideal) would be to overload the services and they can usually be safely observed for some months. Profuse or repeated haemoptysis (however slight), whether with or without radiological abnormalities or physical signs, should, however, always lead to bronchoscopy: a variety of bronchial abnormalities may be found confirming a diagnosis or indicating appropriate further investigation (see Chapter 10 and Plates 55, 64, 65, 84, 96, 132, 154, 170, 174 & 179). It must be stressed that bronchoscopy should not be delayed because the patient is actually bleeding: quite large quantities of blood can be removed with good sucking facilities (Plate 197). If the investigation is delayed an opportunity of assessing the true situation or locating the source may be lost. Nor should the cessation of bleeding deter the bronchoscopist: otherwise silent, but extensive, pathology may still be found in a large bronchus (Plates 150, 199 & 200). Furthermore, the routine use of the bronchofibrescope will sometimes reveal a small lesion in a segmental or subsegmental bronchus which not only has stopped bleeding but has failed to produce other clinical or radiological signs.

Cough, wheeze, stridor and dyspnoea

Cough of recent onset, unexplained and persistent, with or without sputum, must always raise the suspicion of a bronchial lesion, a foreign body, or bronchial distortion (Plates 86, 113, 166, 203, 206 & 232). Less well recognised, however, is the significance of a *change in cough habit* which is frequently missed in chronic bronchitics, with their already long history of cough and sputum. Bronchial carcinoma not infrequently presents in this way (Plates 118, 154, 162 & 199).

Wheeze, either in the patient's story, or found on examination, carries a similar significance to cough when it is of recent onset and persistent. Of particular importance is a *unilateral wheeze which will not disappear on coughing* or, if it does, *always returns to the same place*: such a finding is diagnostic of bronchial narrowing (Plates 98, 102, 106, 135, 140 & 157). Stridor heard over the largest airways is similarly significant (Plates 97, 136, 211 & 220): it is discussed further in Chapter 10.

Dyspnoea, also, can be associated with visible pathology in the bronchial tree. It most often occurs with other symptoms, particularly related to lymphangitis carcinomatosa (Plate 143) or bronchial obstruction. This obstruction may be either partial, together with wheeze, cough or other symptom (Plates 136, 141, 157, 174,

175 & 220); or complete, together with signs of pulmonary collapse (Plate 195). Occasionally, dyspnoea may be the lone presenting abnormality in a patient with a bronchoscopically visible lesion (Plates 165 & 168).

Aspiration

The possibility of an aspirated foreign body, vomit or blood, particularly in children, must never be forgotten when taking the history. Although adult patients sometimes have absolutely no memory of a 'choking' episode (Plate 216) and so may mislead the physician, foreign bodies are far more frequently not included in the differential diagnosis because of the physician's own inattention to detail. Cough of recent onset, associated with choking or holding objects in the mouth, or after anaesthesia, accident, alcoholic stupor or vomiting, is of great clinical significance. Wheeze may occur immediately, or follow if oedema develops. Purulent sputum and pyrexia may occur as infection supervenes (Plate 215). Haemoptysis is not uncommon. Bronchoscopy is urgent on suspicion: to delay is to risk lung abscess, or other dangerous infection, and increasing oedema, which will make the removal of the foreign object or material very much more difficult and hazardous. Occasionally, provided the foreign body does not occlude a bronchus completely, it may produce only minor symptoms and remain almost harmlessly in situ for many years (Plates 217 & 218).

If aspiration occurs due to swallowing problems or from a lesion in the proximal bronchial tree itself, pulmonary abscess may follow or multiple repeated pneumonias may appear in different pulmonary segments. Bronchoscopy can often elucidate such cases (Plates 61, 131 & 178).

Bronchial obstruction

Certain syndromes, in addition to aspiration, may suggest bronchial obstruction, but do not indicate the cause, leaving bronchoscopy as the most useful diagnostic aid. Signs of pulmonary collapse, either segmental, lobar or whole lung (Plates 62, 68, 149, 154, 165, 166, 195, 198, 201 & 202), obstructive overinflation (Plate 157), repeated infections in the same area of lung (Plates 94, 160 & 171) and pneumonia that does not clear satisfactorily with antimicrobial treatment (Plates 67 & 114) are the most important syndromes. Cough, with or without sputum and possibly with wheeze, may accompany any of them.

A situation that needs special mention is that of postoperative pulmonary collapse and infection. Usually this is not due to aspiration of infected material unless anaesthesia has been administered in an emergency. The condition more often develops in patients who were already producing sputum before operation and who find coughing both difficult and painful thereafter. Physiotherapy is frequently inadequate, but bronchial toilet via the bronchoscope can produce a dramatic change (Plate 60).

Radiological changes

Persistent or recurrent pneumonia, and segmental, lobar or pulmonary collapse,

5

often diagnosed radiologically, have been mentioned above as part of the syndromes of bronchial obstruction. They are the commonest causes of radiological abnormalities indicating bronchoscopy. Associated with these, or found alone, may be the typical enlarged hilar shadow so common in bronchial carcinoma (Plates 97 & 163). Any other shadow suggesting intrathoracic lymphadenopathy is also an indication: not only may the diagnosis be obtained by transbronchial aspiration biopsy of the lymph nodes themselves (Plate 106) but intrabronchial lesions can often be found that were not visible, or suspected, radiographically (Plates 86, 204, 206, 216 & 217). Local overinflation of pulmonary tissue, suggesting partial bronchial obstruction and consequent air trapping, should also lead to bronchoscopy (Plate 157).

A more peripheral shadow suggesting a mass, particularly if persistent, rounded or enlarging, should always be considered to represent a tumour until proved otherwise. Patients with such lesions are commonly not considered for bronchoscopy because the causal pathology is expected to be beyond vision and percutaneous fine needle aspiration is more likely to provide a diagnosis. This, however, is a specious argument. Not only may the tumour have grown proximally along a bronchus (Plates 164, 166 & 167) but much information can be obtained via the bronchoscope without a view of the presumed tumour itself. The segmental bronchus involved can be inspected for secondary invasion, secretions may be obtained for cytology and, with miniature forceps or brush thrust peripherally via the fibrescope (with radiographic control if necessary), tumour material may often be obtained. Furthermore, it may become evident that there is local node enlargement, indicating metastic involvement, which was not visible radiologically (Plate 117). Finally, negative findings are themselves of value in determining further investigations or treatment alternatives.

Radiological changes suggesting pulmonary abscess (Plate 61), whether or not accompanied by the clinical features of aspiration described above, should always lead to bronchoscopy. Some patients are relatively symptomless but may have an underlying carcinoma.

Now that transbronchial pulmonary biopsy is a routine procedure, bronchoscopy also may be indicated in cases of diffuse pulmonary shadowing where the diagnosis has not been obtained by other means. Bronchial mucosal biopsy may also give the diagnosis in some cases, for example miliary tuberculosis, lymphangitis carcinomatosa and sarcoidosis (Plates 82, 143, 205 & 206).

Diagnosis of pulmonary infection

The bronchoscope has a most useful role to play when it is proving difficult to establish the cause of a respiratory infection, particularly in an immunocompromised person; an increasing problem in patients with HIV infection. A variety of infective organisms (for example *Pneumocystis carinii*, cytomegalovirus. *Aspergillus* and the tubercle bacillus) can, in such patients, cause serious infection without sputum, expressed sputum, or other specimens being adequate for diagnosis. Secretions, washings from bronchoalveolar lavage, and lung biopsy specimens, often yield vital information. Unfortunately negative findings

6

by no means exclude such diagnoses and open lung biopsy may still be required. Various catheter designs for collecting specimens free of upper airway contamination are available and are essential if anaerobic infections are to be confidently diagnosed.

The diagnosis of pulmonary tuberculosis, even in an otherwise healthy individual, can also be extremely difficult. Secretions or washings obtained bronchoscopically can be diagnostic and the investigation is well worth undertaking in such circumstances (Plate 84).

Miscellaneous thoracic indications

The cause of a pleural effusion often is ascertained from the fluid itself, from the pleural biopsy or from other clinical features. In a proportion of cases, however, there will be difficulty and, since pleural effusion is a common presenting feature of bronchial carcinoma, bronchoscopy is indicated (Plate 168). Pleuritic pain without fluid may have similar implications (Plates 117 & 141).

In the elderly, active pulmonary tuberculosis can represent a relapse of old disease precipitated by the growth of a carcinoma in the scarred area: this must always be suspected in a heavy smoker and particularly if there is a poor response to anti-tuberculosis chemotherapy (Plate 161).

Very useful information can be obtained in cases of suspected bronchiectasis. Various intrabronchial changes may strongly support the diagnosis and a carcinoma, or forgotten foreign body can be excluded (Plates 63 to 65, 96, 123 to 125). In addition, selective bronchograms can be performed via the bronchoscope.

Severe trauma may well be an indication, particularly if associated with thoracic damage or loss of consciousness, to investigate for possible bronchial rupture or aspiration of foreign material.

Clearly the finding of malignant cells in a patient's sputum is an absolute indication, regardless of whether signs or radiographic changes are present (Plate 145). Even when the diagnosis is established cytologically, bronchoscopy may still give much additional information affecting the choice and details of treatment. Meticulous use of the bronchofibrescope may be particularly rewarding in this circumstance and reveal only a small peripheral tumour, potentially resectable.

Either dysphagia or persistent central, thoracic pain, aching in nature (Plate 97), may be a manifestation of mediastinal spread of bronchial carcinoma. Occasionally either may be the presenting feature.

Extrathoracic indications

Various extrathoracic manifestations, if otherwise unexplained and even if lone signs, should lead to bronchoscopy. This may reveal a carcinoma or other major illness as the primary cause of the changes seen. Examples of such signs are lymph node enlargements in the neck or axillae; unexplained erythema nodosum (Plate 203); superior vena caval obstruction (Plate 136); hypertrophic pulmonary osteoarthropathy and/or finger clubbing, particularly if the nails are tobacco stained (Plates 112 & 164); neuromyopathies (Plate 153); endocrine disturbances, for example inappropriate ADH secretion; gynaecomastia; and voice changes due to involvement of the left recurrent laryngeal nerve in intrathoracic disease (Plates 8, 98, 99, 152 & 163). The isolated finding of cerebral metastases in a smoker should also lead to bronchoscopy, since the finding of an oat-cell carcinoma means that a worthwhile response to chemotherapy may be obtained.

Conclusion

It is clear that the indications for bronchoscopy are many and varied. Almost any puzzling pulmonary condition should be considered for this investigation for *surprises are frequent and the diagnostic yield high. Bronchoscopy should be considered readily and performed without long discussions or delay.*

CHAPTER 3

FIBREOPTIC BRONCHOSCOPY

Introduction

The flexible fibreoptic bronchoscope has made a great impact on the practice of respiratory medicine. Prior to its introduction to clinical use in 1967, very few chest physicians performed their own bronchoscopies: bronchoscopy with the rigid apparatus was usually considered a surgical procedure. However, the remarkably low incidence of complications associated with fibroscopy, its ease of use under topical anaesthesia, the fewer people needed at the procedure and its lower cost, have together ensured its worldwide adoption by respiratory physicians. A major advance has been achieved in visualising, and sampling, bronchial pathology very much more peripherally than is possible using rigid telescopes. In addition, nearly all endobronchial procedures can be performed with a fibrescope. Sometimes, however, it is more appropriate and safer to use the rigid bronchoscope because of certain disadvantages inherent in the fibrescope which will be discussed later.

The instrument can be inserted in various ways; via the nose, the mouth, endotracheal or tracheostomy tubes, or through the rigid bronchoscope. In the hands of the skilled and sympathetic operator, using the fibrescope alone and topical anaesthesia, patient acceptance is good. However, the apparent simplicity and safety of the procedure should not allow the uninformed operator, who has experience of fibreoscopy alone, to assume that there are no dangers, or that rigid bronchoscopy no longer has a role to play. A well-trained respiratory physician is able to pass either instrument skilfully and employ the complementary attributes of the two methods.

The various techniques for anaesthetising the airway, and subsequently inserting the fibrescope, each have their advocates, but the very persistence of these varying techniques indicates that many are equally acceptable: each bronchoscopist will find a preferred method. This section describes only those techniques most commonly used: no attempt is made to describe a *best* method.

Preparing the patient

The best, and essential, preparation of the patient is careful and sympathetic explanation of what a bronchoscopy entails, followed by a second, careful, step-by-step

9

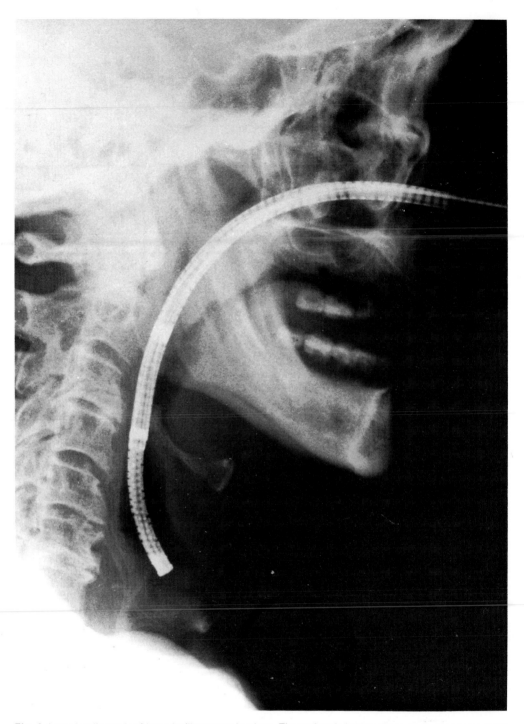

Fig. 1 Lateral radiograph of bronchofibrescope in place. The patient is in the sitting posture and the nasal approach has been chosen. The route through the inferior meatus, behind the tongue, posterior to the epiglottis, and past the hyoid bone, so that the tip lies just beyond the larynx and approaches the partially calcified cricoid cartilage, is well seen. (Taken by the X-Ray Department, Churchill Hospital, Oxford.)

explanation at the time of the procedure. The patient must know that there is no danger, that the local anaesthetic will prevent pain and that concentrating on relaxed breathing will greatly facilitate the examination. Furthermore, he should be warned of the most unpleasant taste of the anaesthetic, of the urge to cough and of the dysphonia which will follow passing the fibrescope through the glottis. Without these preliminaries, the operator is unlikely to gain the patient's full and relaxed cooperation. Using this technique, some bronchoscopists are able to dispense with sedatives without reducing the patient's acceptance, topical anaesthesia alone proving adequate. Acceptability probably depends more on rapport, and therefore on the temperaments of patient and operator, than on any other factor.

Premedication

If premedication is to be used, atropine (0.6–1.2 mg, injected intramuscularly 30–40 minutes before operating) is often advised to prevent vasovagal events and reduce secretions. However, such events are very unlikely in the supine position and secretions usually can be aspirated. Opiates, for example alfentanil, help to suppress cough, as well as anxiety, and, in the event of excessive respiratory depression, can be reversed with intravenous naloxone. Short-acting benzodiazepines (for example midazolam) relieve anxiety and provide a degree of amnesia for the procedure. In addition, any respiratory depression can be reversed with flumazenil.

Positioning the patient

Most operators prefer to face the semi-recumbent or sitting patient throughout the procedure (Figure 2); others stand at the head of the supine patient (Figure 3). An alternative is to change his position from sitting to lying when the most critical phase of the operation has passed; either after instillation of the local anaesthetic or when the bronchoscope reaches the pharynx.

Lying semi-recumbent on the examination couch, with its head end raised to an angle of 45° is not a very comfortable or stable posture. There is little support for the lower back and the patient tends to slide down the couch unless an adjustable foot board is provided: a more upright sitting posture may be more comfortable. Lying supine is even more comfortable and the patient is least likely to suffer vaso-vagal attacks. Furthermore, the bronchoscope does not have to be held at the oper-ator's shoulder level during the procedure. The situation is, arguably, more relaxed for both patient and bronchoscopist. It is, nevertheless, wise to protect the recum-bent patient's eyes from accidental injury; but this may generate anxiety.

Alternatively, a sitting patient provides face-to-face contact throughout, pre-ferred by most operators, as well as making it very much easier for the patient to cough.

The spacial orientation of the bronchial tree clearly depends on where the oper-ator stands in relation to the patient. However, he should be able to view the tree from any angle if he understands the anatomy thoroughly and thinks in three dimensions.

Precautions

Before proceeding one should check that the patient has received any prescribed premedication and followed instructions to avoid food and drink for, at least, three hours: gagging is quite common and the occasional vomiting particularly hazardous when the larynx is anaesthetised.

Resuscitative drugs and apparatus, including a rigid bronchoscope, should be available and regularly checked. Since biopsies are usually taken, any doubt about the patient's haemostasis should have led to investigation and appropriate corrective precautionary measures.

Patients with significant hypoxaemia should receive additional oxygen by nasal catheter. Potentially dangerous, additional hypoxaemia (with or without bronchospasm) can be induced by lignocaine, prolonged coughing, bronchoalveolar lavage or simply passing the fibrescope. Monitoring of arterial oxygen saturation by pulse oximetry is recommended if there is any doubt about the patient's oxygenation.

Patients with asthma should receive 5 mg of nebulised salbutamol prior to bronchoscopy to avoid a serious increase in bronchospasm. Further salbutamol should be available, in case required during or after the procedure.

Finally, protection of the operator should be considered. Transmission of infection from patient to operator is highly unlikely, but possible. Such transmission could be by droplet inhalation, conjunctival innoculation or through minor abrasions or cuts on the hands. Hepatitis B and BCG vaccination should be firmly recommended to all bronchoscopists, but HIV transmission can only be guarded against by barrier methods. Hence the current recommendation is that, even if there is only the slightest possibility that the patient could be HIV positive, then a theatre gown, theatre cap, mask, goggles and rubber gloves should all be worn.

Topical anaesthesia

Although some operators still use cocaine for its greater effectiveness, lignocaine (2–4%) is considered much safer and is the most widely used agent. It can be used as a spray from a hand atomiser or pressurised aerosol container, in finer particles from a nebuliser, or in gel form. It is usually advised that a total of 400 mg should not be exceeded (20 ml of 2% solution) but, in practice, more is sometimes required. This appears safe, probably because a proportion is expectorated immediately.

It is stressed again that, while applying topical anaesthesia for either nasal or oral intubation, full and sympathetic information and reassurance must be given continuously to ensure the patient's confidence and relaxation. There should be no hurry to proceed and time must always be allowed for maximum anaesthesia to develop *after each application* (2–3 minutes): a painful introduction to the procedure will rapidly destroy the patient's confidence. In particular, it must be remembered that topical anaesthesia only abolishes surface sensation; pressure, especially on the nasal turbinates, remains very uncomfortable, or even painful. The most gentle manoeuvring is all that is possible.

The nose is exquisitely sensitive and passing the bronchoscope through a small nasal passage often is the most unpleasant part of the whole procedure. Nevertheless, this route often is preferred to the mouth because the patient can cough more comfortably and the fibrescope cannot be bitten. However, even if the most patent nasal passage is chosen, as indicated by the patient or by direct inspection, it sometimes proves too small for the larger fibrescopes and the mouth has to be used.

Varying degrees of mucosal anaesthesia can be obtained in the nose either by inhaling lignocaine solution from a nebuliser, by spraying with a hand atomiser directly into the nasal passages, or by introducing lignocaine gel. Standard nebulisers produce particles that deposit in the small airways. Minor modification to the apparatus can produce the preferred larger particles which, when inhaled through the mouth or nose, begin to anaesthetise the upper airway. Some success has also been reported using ultrasonically nebulised lignocaine (for example from a De Vilbiss 35B nebuliser). Such nebulisers are capable of quickly delivering very large and potentially toxic quantities of lignocaine throughout the bronchial tree: 10 ml of 4% solution has proved safe.

Pressurised lignocaine sprays often produce extreme discomfort and even sinus pain when used in the nose, probably because of sudden increase in intranasal pressure: they are best reserved for use beyond the turbinates or via the mouth. Lignocaine gel, gently squeezed into the nose until tasted in the nasopharynx, is much more comfortable and extremely effective. It creates no obstruction to subsequent passage of the fibrescope, which, if necessary, can easily be achieved by feel rather than direct vision (see below). Perhaps the commonest method of anaesthetising the nose, however, is spraying with the hand atomiser.

The pressurised spray subsequently can be used to anaesthetise the pharynx and larynx either via the nose (after proceeding as above) or the mouth. Anaesthesia via the nose can be facilitated if the metal applicator provided is replaced by a thin polythene tube of appropriate diameter and flexibility. Its particular advantage lies in allowing atraumatic passage through the already anaesthetised nose, to place the tube tip in the pharynx directed towards the vocal cords. Once this point is reached the patient is asked to protrude his tongue and spraying is synchronised with inspiration. This usually provokes coughing which diminishes with each spray if 2 minutes is allowed between them: preparation is complete when coughing is no longer provoked.

If the peroral route is employed the pressurised spray provides adequate topical anaesthesia. The sitting posture is comfortable for the patient and convenient for the operator. The patient's shoulders should be fully relaxed and the chin jutted forward, so making the glottis as accessible as possible. The tongue is protruded and held forward while the oropharynx, back of the tongue and entrance to the larynx are sprayed progressively, and synchronously with inspirations.

An alternative technique, increasingly used, is to inject quickly about 5 ml of 2% or 4% lignocaine through the cricothyroid membrane. This produces a paroxysm of coughing which effectively distributes the lignocaine both upwards and downwards to anaesthetise the vocal cords and proximal bronchial tree. A 23 gauge 'butterfly' infusion needle allows fast injection with minimal trauma. The needle should be removed quickly after the injection is completed to reduce

13

the chance that the coughing spasm might drive it into the wall of trachea or larynx: a 'butterfly' needle is safer than a plain needle since it can move more freely with the gross movements of the whole larynx.

Final complete anaesthesia of the larynx is achieved, as necessary, by gently trickling lignocaine through the fibrescope operating channel onto the cords until no further immediate coughing results (see 'Negotiating the larynx' below).

Pernasal insertion

Having waited for effective local anaesthesia, the tip of the bronchoscope is passed through the chosen nostril. The shaft can be lubricated with lignocaine gel if this has not already been used in the nose. The largest passage is the inferior meatus, below the inferior turbinate, along the floor of the nose. This route should be followed by *passing the fibrescope directly backwards, not obliquely upwards* (Figs 1 & 2). Often it is best gently to feel one's way through the nose, but direct vision may be preferred.

Control of the instrument is best achieved by keeping the whole length of the shaft *as straight as possible*, one hand on the control and the other steadying the shaft: the tip is more accurately and predictably responsive to movements of the control in these circumstances. A slight caudal deflection of the tip will help to keep the instrument in the inferior meatus.

As the back of the nose is reached, the fibrescope tip should be angled much more caudally (about 60°–80°) to pass through the nasopharynx into the space

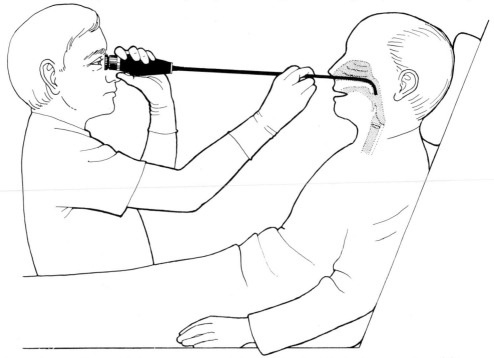

Fig. 2 Pernasal fibreoptic bronchoscopy in the sitting position. Keeping the fibrescope as straight as possible, the tip is passed directly backwards through the inferior meatus and into the nasopharynx. Here, caudal deflection has provided the view shown in Plate 2. (Compare Fig. 1.)

behind the tongue (Figs 1 & 2). According to the relative positions of the patient and operator, one now obtains either the view illustrated in Plate 1 (operator behind supine patient) or that in Plate 2 (operator facing sitting patient).

It is easy to get lost in the folds of the posterior nasopharyngeal wall, but keeping the fibrescope shaft straight and aligned with the inferior meatus, maintaining adequate flexion of the tip and asking the patient to protrude the tongue will all help. If lignocaine gel was used, the objective lens may be obscured: it can now be cleansed by wiping on the mucosa.

If the nasal passage first chosen cannot be negotiated by gentle manipulation (blood drawn is a sign of failure!), the other can be tried following appropriate anaesthesia. Failing this, the operator must change to peroral insertion.

Peroral insertion

When using the oral route either the sitting or supine (Fig. 3) posture may be used. It is important to ensure that the back of the tongue was included in the anaesthesia. An annular bite guard is threaded over the fibrescope and held in readiness near the control head. The patient now opens his mouth and protrudes the tongue: this may be held protruded by the patient or an assistant, as appropriate.

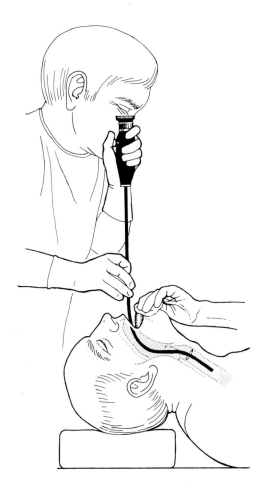

The fibrescope is introduced as far as the back of the tongue and the tip is then deflected caudally by 50°–60°. This should allow a view similar to that obtained via the nose (Plate 1 or 2). The bite guard should now be threaded down the fibrescope shaft and placed in position. Only as the bite guard is about to be inserted should the tongue be released and further progress attempted: an accidental bite can ruin a fibrescope.

Fig. 3 Peroral fibreoptic bronchoscopy in the supine position. The fibrescope is kept as straight as possible. The tongue is protruded and pulled forward by the patient or an assistant. This prevents closure of the mouth and facilitates location of the epiglottis via the oropharynx. The bite guard has been omitted for simplicity.

Negotiating the larynx

Once the larynx is in view, vocal cord movement must be studied during phonotion and the pharynx, epiglottis and cords inspected for abnormalities, particularly tumours (Plates 7–10). Before negotiating the glottis, adequacy of anaesthesia must be investigated by gently trickling lignocaine solution on to the cords. Forceful squirting of the anaesthetic on to sensitive cords should be avoided, as this can be distressing. If coughing is provoked (the patient should be warned of this possibility) 2 minutes must pass before more lignocaine is applied. This procedure should be repeated until no immediate response is obtained.

The patient must now be warned that he or she will become hoarse, but that the voice will return immediately the procedure is over. During a quiet inspiration the fibrescope is passed slowly and very gently through the glottis. If this causes coughing, there should be immediate withdrawal from the cords and more anaesthetic applied: the sequence is repeated as necessary until the cords are negotiated without response.

Other methods of insertion

If it is decided to introduce an endotracheal tube, when operating through the mouth, the most meticulous care will be needed when applying the topical anaesthesia: patients are much less tolerant of a wide tube than of the fibrescope alone. Some operators block the superior laryngeal nerves, in addition to carrying out the routine described above. This is done by using long curved forceps to apply a swab, soaked in 4% lignocaine, to each pyriform fossa for at least 1 minute. Others use a laryngeal mirror to ensure accurate placing of the lignocaine solution under direct vision. This technique renders blocking of the superior laryngeal nerves unnecessary and in skilful hands is probably the most acceptable to the patient. The fibrescope is introduced in the same way as already outlined under 'Peroral insertion', but with the endotracheal tube replacing the bite guard. Once the fibrescope is in the trachea, the tube can gently be insinuated through the glottis by threading it down the shaft and then be kept in place for the duration of the procedure with adhesive tape.

In the intensive care situation the fibrescope can be extremely useful either for diagnostic purposes or to remove accumulated secretions. A tube, either endotracheal or tracheostomy, is usually already in situ and the instrument can be inserted easily provided the tube is of adequate diameter. Alternatively the fibrescope can be introduced alongside a smaller endotracheal tube, with the cuff temporarily deflated to allow its passage. However, in some circumstances the fibrescope will prove inadequate (for example for the removal of inhaled foreign bodies or the very tenacious secretions that may be found in such patients): the indwelling tube will have to be temporarily removed to allow insertion of a rigid bronchoscope (Plates 223 & 224).

A few fibreoscopists prefer to operate with general anaesthesia. A standard cuffed endotracheal tube is introduced and one of various available adapters added to allow closed circuit inhalation anaesthesia with the fibrescope in situ. The oxygen Venturi technique, associated with intravenous anaesthesia, can also be applied in this situation and has its advantages. The internal diameter of the tube must be at least 8.5 mm to allow adequate ventilation when the usual 5 or 5.5 mm bronchofibrescope is in place. It is suggested, however, that once a general anaesthetic has been chosen the logic is to use a *straight* tube with its attendant advantages.

Examining the bronchial tree

Once past the glottis, whichever route and method of anaesthesia was chosen, 2% lignocaine solution should be adequate and can be sprayed as necessary via the aspirating channel. Patients vary considerably in sensitivity: some need further anaesthetic solution only when the upper bronchi are entered, others 2 ml each to trachea, carina, main bronchi, upper bronchial orifices and the site of any biopsy. The quantity required will be minimised if the operator maintains gentleness and patience, avoids touching bronchial walls wherever possible and responds immediately to slight coughing: once severe it is difficult to control. The supine position has the advantage of tending to keep anaesthetic and instrument together on the posterior bronchial walls.

Before proceeding, the bronchoscopist must understand the limitations of anatomical knowledge. At the more peripheral level reached by the fibrescope, individual bronchial orifices or branches cannot be recognised by their configuration; they are all too similar and variations are common. *One's position in the peripheral bronchial tree can only be appreciated by knowing how one got there.* Furthermore, the operator must continually think of the bronchial tree in three-dimensional terms: this becomes particularly important when handling the fibrescope in narrow, branching passages where its remarkable directional abilities make it easy to lose one's way. Withdrawing to the carina for reorientation helps in these circumstances.

The examination is carried out in a methodical, routine fashion to ensure that nothing is missed, taking care not to traverse the trachea too quickly and thus fail to see the rare lesions that may occur in this region. The inspection of orifices in a strict order avoids missing one and leads either to their accurate identification or to the recognition of their absence, or to the discovery of supernumerary bronchi. Any deviation or distortion and the type, location and quantity of any secretion present should be carefully noted. Secretion must be *delicately* removed by sucker to avoid damage and obscuration by bleeding (see Chapter 9): the condition and colour of the mucosa can then be observed. Any additional lesion must be carefully examined and, finally, specimens may be taken for cytology and histology. This routine should be followed throughout the bronchial tree. It is a good plan to examine last the side which is likely to be abnormal, for any investigation (particularly biopsy) can produce bleeding which may well interfere with any further examination.

Manipulating the fibrescope

It is important to realise that manipulating the bronchofibrescope is very much more difficult than would seem at first sight. The novice must be prepared for some frustrating experiences and not lose heart. The only answer is considerable manipulative practice. This is not obtained easily or quickly under clinical conditions and therefore practice with a lung model is strongly recommended: the appropriate flexing and/or rotatory movements for directing the movable tip in the desired direction eventually become almost automatic. Thus, since learning to use the bronchofibrescope is essentially practice, verbal descriptions can give only an outline of the procedure. What follows can indicate, only briefly, the most important practical points.

The various makes and models of bronchofibrescope available will not be discussed here: they are all designed on the same principle and incorporate a directable tip controlled from the head of the instrument. Familiarity with the controls only comes with the practice already recommended. Suffice it to say that they are extremely expensive, delicate instruments and must be handled with the utmost care. Forced angulation can damage the guide wires, fibre bundles or both. Even under operating conditions, with the instrument within the bronchial tree, it is not difficult to damage the control mechanism. Forced twisting or flexing must never be attempted when the tip is in a narrow orifice, nor must the instrument be removed without assisting the tip to return to the neutral position as it gradually retreats along the possibly tortuous course already taken. Never withdraw a fibrescope with the control in the 'locked' position. A sensitive response to the small forces transmitted to the operator's fingers is mandatory to avoid damage to the apparatus or to the patient.

The instrument should only be inserted after adjusting the tip to the neutral, forward-viewing position. The best hold for the individual operator and instrument will have been discovered during practice, but it is recommended that a 'one hand' hold and thumb control be developed whenever possible, using the left hand. This not only leads to economy of movement but leaves the right hand free to guide the fibrescope and manipulate accessory instruments—forceps, curette, brush or aspirating tube—without the suction tube or lighting cable getting in the way. By appropriate angulation of the tip and/or rotation of the instrument the whole circumference of the bronchus to be negotiated must be kept constantly in view. Appropriate slight adjustments of angulation and rotation are made to retain this view, and so avoid scraping the bronchial wall as the fibrescope is gently advanced. Cough and bleeding are reduced by this technique and remarkably sharp turns can be negotiated; with practice, most bronchi large enough to admit the instrument can be entered. In difficult, distal situations, advantage can also be taken of respiratory movements to reorientate or slightly advance the fibrescope. Never use force to twist or advance the instrument: the field of view is such that the tip may be snugly fitting a bronchus before this is appreciated by the operator. Again, tactile sensation is at a premium.

Secretions that are not too tenacious can be removed, as necessary, through the aspirating/operating channel of the instrument and usually without soiling the objective lens. Caution and great gentleness are necessary to avoid trauma that may precipitate bleeding and obscure vision; particularly likely when approaching bronchial tumours. For convenience a sucking tube can be left attached during the procedure and brought into operation as necessary. Most instruments include an aspirating port for attachment to a vacuum source; this can be operated by closing a side hole with a finger whilst still allowing insertion of operating instruments. If this facility is not provided, a y-shaped connecting tube can be inserted into the suction channel with the oblique arm connected to the vacuum source. This leaves the straight arm available for instrumentation, or closure with a finger to obtain suction as required. Irrigation with small quantities of normal saline solution injected down the aspirating channel, immediately followed by aspiration, can often clear moderately thick secretions or small quantities of blood.

In some cases blood or secretions will be profuse or tenacious enough to soil the objective lens, block the aspirating channel, or both. If irrigation down the channel, asking the patient to cough, or wiping the objective lens on the mucosa fails to restore clear vision, the fibrescope must be removed and cleaned before proceeding. This may be necessary a number of times: it will certainly be necessary if blood is allowed to clot on the lens or in the aspirating channel.

Specimen taking and the control of bleeding are discussed in Chapter 9.

Disadvantages

The advantages of the fibrescope are obvious, but the potential disadvantages and possible complications of fibreoscopy should be considered carefully, for often they are minimised or not appreciated.

The view obtained with the bronchofibrescope, excellent in most cases, is easily obscured. Although wiping the instrument tip on the bronchial mucosa, or irrigation via the sucking channel, usually clears the lens, removal for cleansing may be necessary and repeated reinsertion can be tedious and uncomfortable for the patient. Furthermore, some secretions, particularly those found in asthmatics or postoperative pulmonary collapse, are very thick and tenacious: they will often defy removal via the narrow channel available (Plates 57 & 62).

It is not possible to feel rigidity of the bronchial tree; this can be sensed easily with a rigid tube or forceps.

Foreign body removal is limited, although some objects may be extracted with specially designed forceps, claw, basket or balloon.

Most importantly, the control of significant haemorrhage, caused by instrumentation, may prove impossible. Vision is rapidly obscured and sucking facilities are limited, making application of control methods very difficult (see Chapter 9).

An attempt to insert a rigid tube, to discover and control the bleeding point, may well fail or not be achieved in time, because of the patient's resistance, obscured vision, lack of training or because the instrument is not available. Furthermore, without a tube in place, ventilation, and resuscitation if necessary, will be very difficult or impossible.

Finally, in bronchitic patients, and even more so in patients with tight tracheal strictures, blood gases can be deranged simply by passing the fibrescope alone, in contradistinction to the safe situation achieved with oxygen Venturi ventilation down a rigid tube.

These limitations are only relative and minor in a statistical sense, but can lead to disaster in the individual case, particularly if the operator, oblivious to their existence, fails to take appropriate precautions and meticulous care.

Cleansing the fibrescope

The advent of hepatitis B and HIV infection has greatly increased concern over bronchoscope disinfection. So much so that many units keep separate fibrescopes for patients with HIV infection. The problem is not completely solved in this way, however, because some patients are unexpectedly HIV positive and others, at high risk, subsequently prove negative. Thus efficient decontaminating procedures are essential and totally immersible fibrescopes mandatory.

Of particular importance is physical cleansing of the fibrescope and its close attachments (sucker assembly, etc) because even prolonged soaking in a disinfectant may not penetrate to the centre of particulate matter. The suction valve should be dismantled and the parts, with the fibrescope, completely immersed in fresh detergent. The equipment must then be thoroughly washed and brushed, including all ports and channels.

The fibrescope and accessories are next left to soak in 2% glutaraldehyde, an agent known to kill all the encountered infecting agents, although the necessary contact time varies considerably: about an hour for mycobacterium tuberculosis; under five minutes for the HIV virus.

This is followed by thorough rinsing with sterile water or 70% alcohol. Any moisture left in the fibrescope allows bacterial colonisation, hence complete drying is essential.

Due to various sensitivity reactions to glutaraldehyde (asthma, dermatitis, conjunctivitis), the ideal system is a closed automatic washer. These units are expensive, but using alternative disinfectants is less satisfactory, either because they are less active against some infecting agents, or because of damage to the fibrescope. Local circumstances will ultimately dictate the actual cleansing protocol.

Following cleansing, the fibrescope is best stored hanging in a tall cupboard with the control head uppermost: repeated replacement and removal from the case provided usually leads to accidental damage during lid closure and to expensive optical repairs.

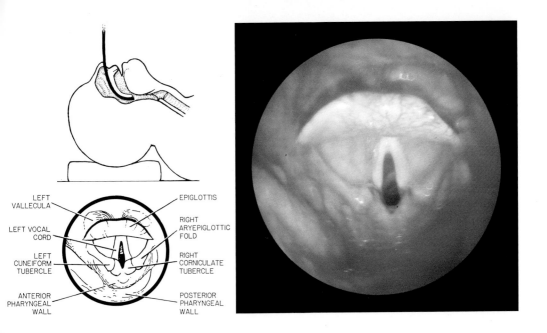

LEFT VALLECULA

EPIGLOTTIS

LEFT VOCAL CORD

RIGHT ARYEPIGLOTTIC FOLD

LEFT CUNEIFORM TUBERCLE

RIGHT CORNICULATE TUBERCLE

ANTERIOR PHARYNGEAL WALL

POSTERIOR PHARYNGEAL WALL

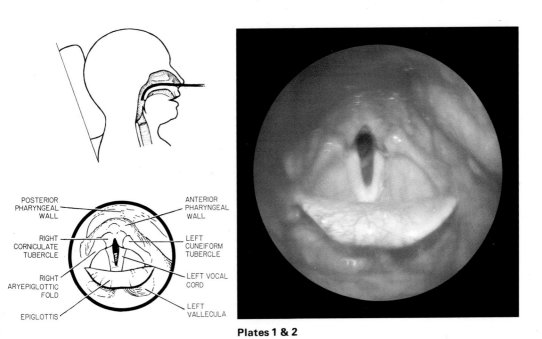

POSTERIOR PHARYNGEAL WALL

ANTERIOR PHARYNGEAL WALL

RIGHT CORNICULATE TUBERCLE

LEFT CUNEIFORM TUBERCLE

RIGHT ARYEPIGLOTTIC FOLD

LEFT VOCAL CORD

LEFT VALLECULA

EPIGLOTTIS

Plates 1 & 2

View of larynx from level of soft palate. This is the view obtained with the fibrescope after traversing the nose and angulating the tip parallel with the posterior pharyngeal wall. The landmarks are clearly seen: the epiglottis proximally, the aryepiglottic folds, and, in the distance, the vocal cords in the relaxed position. Plate 1 shows the view obtained by the bronchoscopist operating behind the supine patient. Plate 2 is that seen by the operator facing the sitting patient.

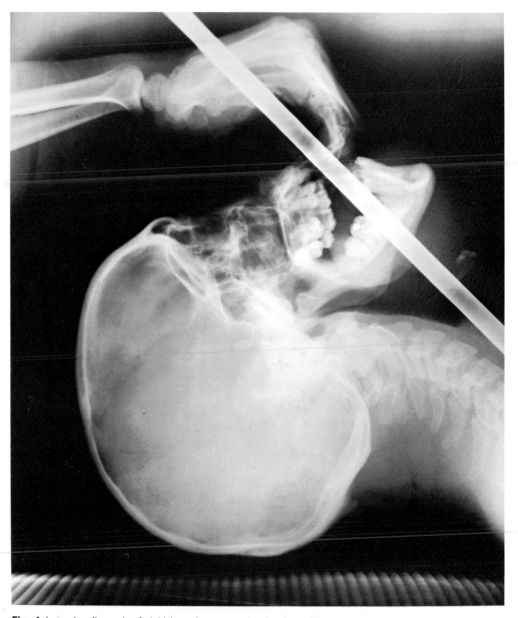

Fig. 4 Lateral radiograph of rigid bronchoscope tube in place. The correct position for the head is well seen: extended and raised some inches from the table. (Taken by the Department of Diagnostic Radiology, Hammersmith Hospital.)

CHAPTER 4

RIGID TUBE BRONCHOSCOPY

Introduction

Ideally, all aspiring bronchoscopists should be trained to use both rigid and flexible apparatus under operating room conditions and thus be equipped for all eventualities. The lone bronchofibreoscopist may occasionally be at a grave disadvantage if faced with a major haemorrhage and has not instant access to the rigid tube and familiarity with its introduction. Furthermore, although passing a fibroscope alone under topical anaesthesia is far less distressing to a patient than introducing a rigid tube under similar conditions (a technique thus made obsolete), it remains true that operating under expertly administered general anaesthesia, together with oxygen Venturi ventilation, is safe and the least unpleasant of all. If these facilities are available, there is no contraindication to a straight rigid tube with its attendant potential advantages.

Potential advantages

A very adequate airway is always present in case resuscitation becomes necessary. Similarly this allows the control of ventilation and blood gases, required in patients with hypoxaemia due to respiratory failure or other causes: thus bronchoscopy becomes possible in such patients.

The management of haemorrhage can well become a major problem during bronchoscopy, but is much more readily controlled if a straight tube is in place (see Chapter 9).

Rigid bronchoscopy should certainly be the first choice if significant haemoptysis is already occurring (Plates 197 & 198), or if it is known preoperatively that there is a risk of haemorrhage. It would even be wise to consider rebronchoscopy with the rigid technique if a vascular central tumour, needing biopsy, is discovered at fibreoscopy: continuous bleeding from a large airway cannot be readily controlled with the fibrescope.

Many foreign bodies (Plates 215 to 218) and large tenacious bronchial plugs, such as those found in asthma (Plate 62) and postoperative pulmonary collapse (Plate 60), can only be removed with appropriate rigid forceps or large bore suckers. Efficient bronchial lavage also requires strong sucking facilities.

Rigid tube bronchoscopy is essential in small children and patients with tracheal

23

narrowing: the fibrescope may obstruct or seriously embarrass the smaller airway (Plate 220).

The rigidity of the carina and bronchial tree, so commonly indicating advanced carcinoma, can readily be appreciated with the forceps or sheath itself: during fibreoscopy, this can only occasionally be suspected by careful observation of respiratory movements.

With the rigid tube in place, and the larger forceps available, it is possible to undertake the endobronchial removal of small benign tumours (Plate 171) or the clearance of sufficient tumour tissue to restablish airways (Plates 195 & 196). The larger specimens obtained at routine biopsy are in themselves an advantage to the histologist.

For those interested, quality photography is possible.

Finally, it will be appreciated that using the fibrescope via the rigid tube eliminates the need for lateral and oblique rigid telescopes and greatly extends the operator's view.

Preparing the patient

Patients should always be prepared for rigid bronchoscopy by full but simple explanation, not only of the general anaesthetia, but of the after-effects of the procedure which may be a little frightening to the uninitiated. Irritating cough, lasting for a few minutes, and occasional expectoration of blood following biopsy, particularly should be mentioned. Soreness of the throat or mouth should not occur if the procedure is done with proper care. Muscle pains, 24–48 hours after using suxemethonium chloride as a relaxant drug, can be distressing but are markedly reduced by using initial small doses of either gallamine triethiodide or d-tubo-curarine during induction. Premedication also may form an important part of the patient's preparation but will vary from centre to centre. It can include atropine, to reduce bronchial secretion and vasovagal problems, but whether a drug to allay anxiety is necessary remains debatable. Many such drugs depress respiration and can cause problems postoperatively. The author uses atropine only and ensures that the patient is conscious and coughing when leaving the theatre.

Anaesthesia and ventilation

Of prime importance is adequate time for careful intubation and complete examination of the bronchial tree: there is no virtue in haste, with the consequent risk of only a superficial inspection, if time can be provided safely. Modern anaesthetic drugs, including intravenous barbiturates and muscle relaxants, provide this time and have made general anaesthesia for bronchoscopy safe and much simpler.

Ventilation adequate for gas exchange must obviously be provided for the paralysed patient. This is achieved by the Sanders oxygen Venturi technique for ventilation during general anaesthesia. A free airway and continuous ventilation is provided safely throughout the procedure, allowing anaesthetist and bronchoscopist to work almost independently: there is no need to interrupt ventilation during sucking or manipulative procedures. This technique is the simplest, cheapest and safest ventilation system yet devised and is such an advance that it replaces all others. (Suitable fitments for this form of ventilation are available from bronchoscope manufacturers.) The major problems of underventilation and inadequate time for full examination, teaching and possibly photography are solved. Thus, general anaesthesia is remarkably safe for rigid bronchoscopy. It is rare to find a patient who is not fit for this form of management. Nevertheless, the bronchoscopist should realise the anaesthetist's problem and be prepared to relinquish *immediately* his claim to the airway if this becomes necessary.

Insertion

For routine rigid bronchoscopy on the supine patient the provision of fully mobile head support is not necessary and all the photographs in this book have been obtained while using a standard operating table with the usual vertically moving headpiece. However, if the introduction of the bronchoscope is to be accomplished easily, it is extremely important to have the head in the correct position. This is achieved quite simply by using a well-filled pillow, or an 8 cm thickness of plastic foam, and then firmly extending the head on it so that the chin points vertically upwards: in fact, the position usually assumed when shaving the chin (Figs 4 & 5). Dentures will, of course, have been removed prior to entering the theatre and the upper teeth or gum and the eyes should be protected by a small dressing towel after retracting the upper lip. The forefinger and thumb of the left hand form a support-ing guide for the bronchoscope and carefully protect the teeth or gums from trauma. Additional care should be exercised if the patient has had conservative dentistry. The other left fingers (from inside the mouth) and the palm (from out-side) hold the upper jaw and control head movements (Fig. 6). Under no circum-stances should the upper teeth or gum be used as a fulcrum to lever the bronchoscope into position.

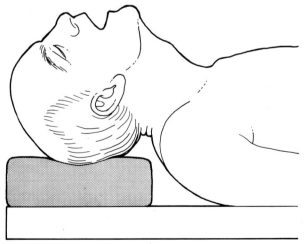

Fig. 5 The patient is anaesthetised and positioned for intubation. The head is resting on a plastic foam pillow to raise it above the table.

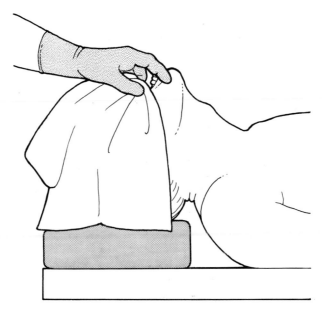

Fig. 6 The upper lip is retracted from the teeth and, after closing the eyes, a protective towel has been positioned in preparation for intubation. The head position is controlled by gripping the maxilla between the palm and last three fingers of the left hand, leaving the forefinger and thumb free to control the instrument. The forefinger should retract the lower lip from the teeth before commencing intubation.

The bronchoscope, previously lubricated for a few centimetres of its distal end only, is held very lightly in the right hand, with its tip uppermost. The actual hold employed will depend upon the design of the instrument. It should be that most calculated not only to retain complete control, but also to be light and sensitive enough to allow reception of tactile impressions from the tip. The instrument is first introduced almost vertically, either (most conveniently) via the right side of the mouth or, in an edentulous patient (more simply), in the midline (Fig. 7). In an anaesthetised patient the tongue forms no obstacle and can easily be pushed forward. However, when performing the instrumentation under topical anaesthesia, no attempt need be made to compress it if this is resisted; instead the instrument can be passed beside the tongue, which then is gently pushed aside.

Occasionally, in an anaesthetised patient, the mouth will not open wide enough for insertion of the tube because the temporomandibular joints do not allow adequate movement of the lower jaw. Such a patient falls into that small group in which the joints are so shaped that a slight posterior movement of the mandible leads to locking: the relaxed jaw in the supine patient naturally takes up this position. The simple remedy is to pull the jaw firmly forward when the mouth will open easily. *Force must not be used.*

As the bronchoscope is inserted further, its proximal end is brought smoothly downwards, using the operator's left thumb as a support. Thus the long axis of the instrument becomes progressively nearer the horizontal as its tip follows the contour of the tongue (Figs. 7 & 8). If this manoeuvre is performed gently, with slight movement of the tip towards the pharynx at the same time, the posterior aspect of the tongue will be reached without trouble and here it should be possible to see the epiglottis (Fig. 8 & Plate 3). The aim now is to gain access to the glottis by passing *posterior* to the epiglottis. Before proceeding further, however, it is important to ensure that the epiglottis and adjacent pharyngeal tissues are normal (Plate 10).

Problems that arise at this stage are usually due to introducing the bronchoscope too rapidly and missing the epiglottis altogether. Occasionally one may pass too anteriorly and so get lost in the spaces between the tongue and epiglottis (epiglottic valleculae). Much more commonly, however, the instrument tip is placed too far posterolaterally. If the landmarks cannot be discovered quickly it is often best partially to withdraw the bronchoscope and try again, more slowly, ensuring that the tip is pointing towards the midline. Aiming at the visible surface prominence of the larynx can ensure this. If this manoeuvre is done slowly and carefully, the epiglottis will be discovered, in the vast majority of cases quite easily, just beyond the root of the tongue. Gentle movement of the bronchoscope tip from side to side and/or lifting it forward by moving the left thumb, will rapidly locate this organ if there is still any difficulty. Under general anaesthesia the epiglottis is sometimes elusive because it can lie on the posterior pharyngeal wall and then it may also be a little difficult to advance further. This can always be managed, however, if care is taken in insinuating the tip of the bronchoscope posterior to the epiglottis and, using the left thumb as a sensitive fulcrum, lifting it gently from the posterior pharyngeal wall.

When this has been achieved it is usually possible immediately to see the posterior part of the laryngeal inlet, with the posterior expansions of the aryepiglottic folds (corniculate tubercles) on either side, and the glottis beyond (Plate 4). The common fault, making this difficult, is again to introduce the bronchoscope too quickly before locating the laryngeal opening, which may be more anterior than expected. The tip may enter the left pyriform fossa, or even oesophagus, and again the answer is partially to withdraw the bronchoscope and reposition it. The secret of finding the larynx easily is to retain a wide angle of view of the area by passing the bronchoscope tip only a *short* way posterior to the epiglottis: just far enough, in fact, to raise this organ without it slipping off the tip of the bronchoscope. Lifting the epiglottis anteriorly, again with the help of the left thumb, will then give a good view of the laryngeal entrance and corniculate tubercles. In a difficult case the anaesthetist can give great help by using gentle external pressure to displace the larynx posteriorly, so making the glottis more accessible. On the rare occasion of great difficulty it may be necessary to expose the glottis with a laryngoscope held in the left hand and then to introduce the bronchoscope with the right.

The loose submucosal tissues of the aryepiglottic folds and corniculate tubercles, and less frequently of the vestibular folds, may hypertrophy to give enlarged fleshy structures that readily fall across the laryngeal inlet in the relaxed, unconscious patient. The glottis may be completely obscured in some cases and it is then necessary to displace these tissues laterally with gentle 'side to side' movements of the bronchoscope tip before access can be gained. In acromegalic patients the hypertrophy can reach formidable proportions making intubation very difficult.

Once the glottis is seen, the bronchoscope can be passed towards it in the midline (Fig 9 & Plate 5). When the cords have been examined carefully to exclude pathological changes (Plates 7 & 9), they should be closely approached with the bronchoscope tube turned through 90°, tip to the right. The axis of the bronchoscope is now directed toward the left vocal cord by centring this in the field of vision and so

27

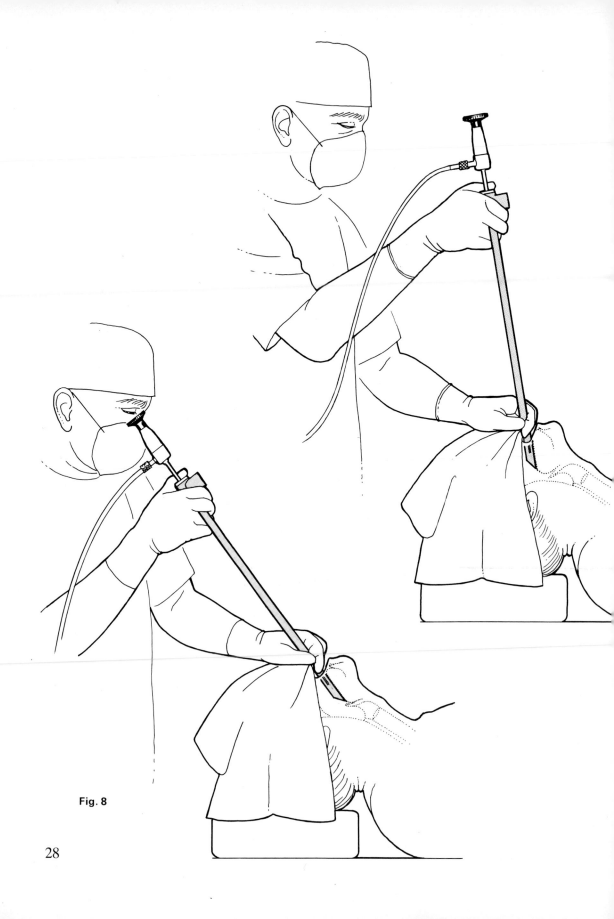

Fig. 8

bringing the tip in line with the glottis (Fig. 10 & Plate 6). Gentle progression will now allow the tip to enter the vertical glottic chink and with a *very careful* twisting movement, associated with further advancement of the bronchoscope, the larynx can be negotiated without trauma. Absolutely no force must be used at this stage: a smaller size of bronchoscope tube may be indicated if there is difficulty. Once through, the normal position of the bronchoscope can be resumed and inspection of the bronchial tree commence (Figs. 11 & 12; Plate 11).

The examination

The first requirement is that the bronchoscope should align with the trachea. Although the head position described is the best for introducing the instrument, it may not be so for further progress. If there is a tendency for the bronchoscope tube to scrape the posterior wall, the position can be corrected by lowering the operating table headpiece: further adjustments, as appropriate, may be necessary during the course of the examination.

If difficulty is experienced in advancing the instrument, in spite of correct align-ment and a visibly clear passage, it is important to check for an external cause: *no force* should be necessary to manipulate a bronchoscope and to use it is dangerous. The tube may be binding on gum or teeth, or be caught in a dental gap. Either the upper or lower lip may not have been adequately retracted from the teeth or gum and so be dragged into the mouth by the advancing bronchoscope tube. Careful lip retraction and placement of the protective towel, together with constant sensitive use of the fingers and thumb of the left hand, will either prevent these problems or immediately sense and correct them on occurrence. Subsequent routine inspection is carried out in the same methodical fashion as described under the heading 'Examining the bronchial tree' in chapter 3.

Positioning of the head and bronchoscope is different for intubating the main and lower bronchi on the two sides and it may also be necessary to alter the head height by adjusting the operating table headpiece. The left side is the more difficult to examine because of the longer, curving course of the main bronchus, and the angle that it makes with the trachea. For examining this side, the bronchoscope is usually and most conveniently kept in the right corner of the mouth while the head

---

Fig. 7 Maintaining the left hand-hold described for Figure 6, the bronchoscope tube is now introduced almost vertically and the tongue displaced forward to allow further insertion. The tip of the instrument is uppermost ready to displace the epiglottis. This principle is the same for all rigid bronchoscopes.*

 * The bronchoscopic sheath illustrated here is a simple tube with Venturi ventilation incorporated. There is no integral light. Consequently all manoeuvres, including intubation, are carried out under telescopic vision. The larger lumen, obtained by discarding integral lighting, was originally determined by the large photographic telescopes then used, but it was soon found that the routine use of telescopes for *all* procedures, including intubation and sucking, carried its own advantages; better vision and accuracy, leading to less traumatic and safer operating. During intubation, the telescope is kept in place by lateral pressure with the right thumb.

Fig. 8 As intubation proceeds the bronchoscope is brought progressively nearer the horizontal until the epiglottis is found, as illustrated here. During this manoeuvre, and continuously throughout the operation, the left thumb and forefinger support and control the instrument to prevent trauma to teeth, gums or lips. (Compare Plate 3.)

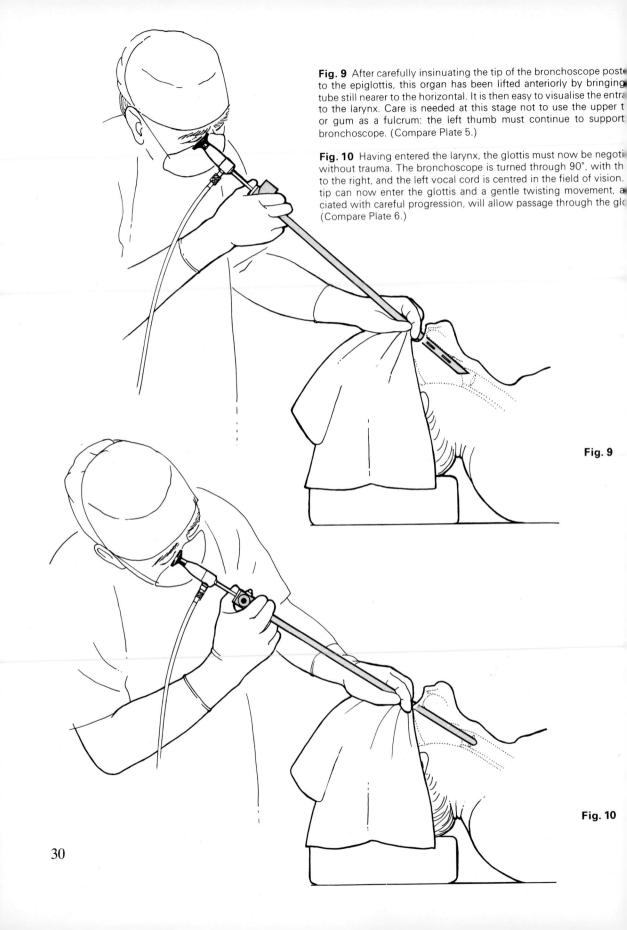

Fig. 9 After carefully insinuating the tip of the bronchoscope post⟨er⟩
to the epiglottis, this organ has been lifted anteriorly by bringing⟨the⟩
tube still nearer to the horizontal. It is then easy to visualise the entra⟨nce⟩
to the larynx. Care is needed at this stage not to use the upper t⟨eeth⟩
or gum as a fulcrum: the left thumb must continue to support ⟨the⟩
bronchoscope. (Compare Plate 5.)

Fig. 10 Having entered the larynx, the glottis must now be negoti⟨ated⟩
without trauma. The bronchoscope is turned through 90°, with th⟨e tip⟩
to the right, and the left vocal cord is centred in the field of vision. ⟨The⟩
tip can now enter the glottis and a gentle twisting movement, a⟨sso⟩
ciated with careful progression, will allow passage through the gl⟨ottis⟩
(Compare Plate 6.)

Fig. 9

Fig. 10

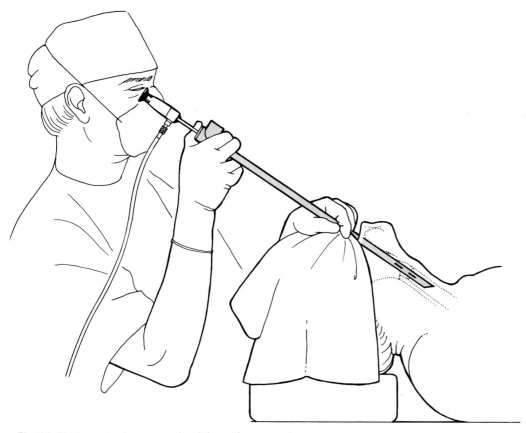

Fig. 11 The larynx has been passed and the trachea entered.

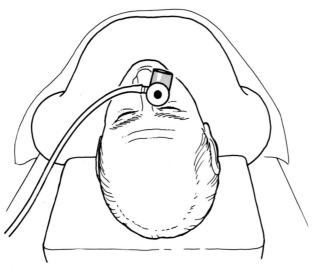

Fig. 12 Bronchoscope tube in trachea. Entry via the right corner of the mouth is illustrated. The head is thus turned very slightly to the left while the tube is in the tracheal axis. The oxygen line to the Venturi injector is seen attached.

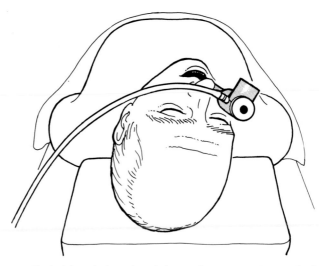

Fig. 13 Bronchoscope tube in left main bronchus. It is usually necessary to turn the head well to the right and to keep the tube in the right corner of the mouth to enter the left main bronchus: a considerable swing to the right is necessary to align bronchoscope and bronchus.

is turned to the right. Thus the proximal end of the tube also swings to the right, allowing its long axis to align with the left main bronchus (Fig. 13). Because of its curved course, further passage down the left main bronchus (and often a view into the upper bronchus) is attained by easing the head and proximal end of the bronchoscope even further to the right as intubation proceeds. Moderate lateral pressure may be needed to obtain correct alignment and safe, nontraumatic intubation. Undue force must *never* be used, either laterally or, even more dangerously, to advance the bronchoscope. When carefully following the described technique the pliancy of the tissues allows passage of the straight tube to a depth in the bronchial tree which at first seems impossible. Nevertheless, because of the curved course of the left main bronchus, its lateral wall is sometimes not clearly seen: an oblique-viewing telescope may be of great value in this situation.

The left lower bronchus usually can be intubated easily, once its orifice is reached, but for a varying distance depending on the size of the patient and the bronchoscope tube used: the primary and even secondary and tertiary divisions of the basal bronchi often can be seen with the best rigid telescopes, which carry their own illumination and are long enough to project well beyond the tube itself. If its origin is suitably oblique, the left upper bronchus also may be entered, or at least well visualised, with the forward-viewing telescope: in these circumstances the division of the lingular bronchus into its superior and inferior branches frequently is seen. Because of great normal variations in the angle of origin, however, a lateral or oblique-viewing telescope may give the best view of the upper bronchus.

The right bronchial tree is the easier to examine, its main and lower bronchi often being a direct continuation of the trachea. Thus, positioning of the bronchoscope or head often is not critical. However, the best view frequently is obtained only by adopting a procedure the reverse of that for the left side: the head is turned to the left with the proximal end of the bronchoscope in the most convenient corner

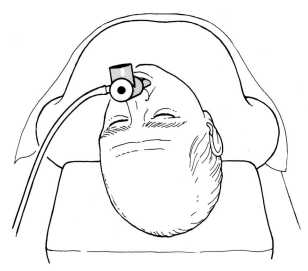

Fig. 14 Bronchoscope tube in right main bronchus. Since the right main bronchus is nearly a continuation of the trachea, the head need only be turned slightly to the left to facilitate further progression. The tube can be kept in the right corner of the mouth and, in fact, it is usual and convenient to use this location only throughout most rigid bronchoscopies.

of the mouth (Fig. 14). An accentuation of this position, using the left corner of the mouth, with the head lowered, may be necessary to obtain the oblique downward and forward view often necessary to see into the middle bronchus. Alternatively it may be found that an oblique or even lateral-viewing telescope may be more suit-

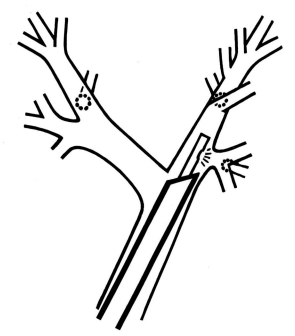

Fig. 15 Use of lateral-viewing telescope. Right upper bronchial orifice. The bronchoscope tube has been positioned as in Figure 14, with the head turned slightly to the left to align trachea and right main bronchus. Accurate alignment and depth of penetration have been determined with forward vision and the lateral-viewing telescope has then been inserted with its objective lens pointing to the right.

able for this orifice. A lateral-viewing telescope is certainly necessary to see into the right upper bronchus, while an oblique or lateral-viewing instrument usually gives the best view of the apical lower bronchi on both sides.

Correct positioning of the lateral-viewing telescope often proves difficult for the beginner: the orifice to be inspected seems very elusive. The first essential is to position the bronchoscope tube appropriately and meticulously by forward vision and carefully to keep it so placed while subsequently manipulating the lateral-viewing telescope (Fig. 15). Branching posterior longitudinal corrugations often will be of value in locating the position of lateral orifices by forward vision (Plate 50). The tube should be inserted to such a depth that the proximal lip of the orifice to be

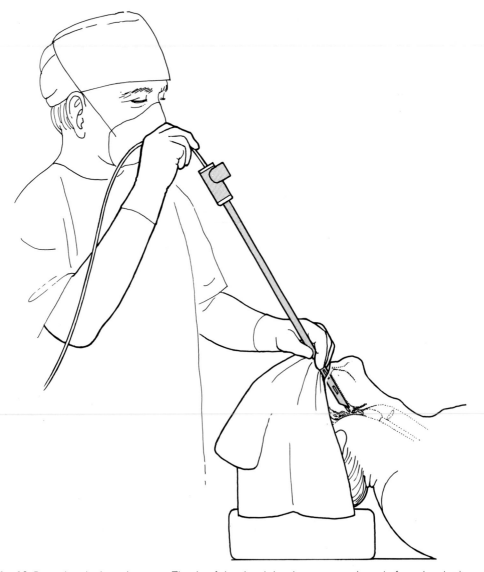

Fig. 16 Removing the bronchoscope. The tip of the sheath has been removed gently from the glottis and now lies in the pharynx. The vocal cords have been inspected for mobility and possible trauma. The operator, after the specimen trap has been removed from the sucker line, is cleansing the pharynx before finally removing the sheath and inspecting lips and teeth, or gums, for possible trauma.

viewed is clearly seen, but only just within the field of forward vision (Plate 15): this not only ensures that the whole orifice will be beyond the tip of the tube and so open to inspection, but also that the depth to which the telescope will have to be inserted will be the same whenever the manoeuvre is practised. The alignment of the tube, in addition to depth of insertion, is also critical: it must be strictly in the long axis of the main bronchus in which it lies. Following these two rules for placing the bronchoscope tube not only ensures that no damage is done by subsequent piston-like movements of the telescope, but that the manoeuvre can be accurately carried out for all orifices, so making them easier to find telescopically. The telescope is now introduced steadily and slowly with the lateral-viewing lens pointing in approximately the correct direction, as determined by an estimate of this from the previous forward view. Directly bronchial mucosa is seen beyond the tip of the tube it is clear that the desired orifice must be nearly in view. Provided the described plan has been followed, only small further movements—piston-like and/or rotary—will now be needed to locate it (Plate 17).

Removal

Removal of the bronchoscope requires care, just as does insertion. This should be done visually until the tube tip reaches the tongue, *not* entirely by feel. The rare protrusion of soft tissue through the lateral ventilation slots will then be spotted immediately. Persistent withdrawal without correcting this accident can produce a dangerous guillotine effect. The lips, gums or teeth should continue to be protected with the left hand, so that as the instrument is gently withdrawn it cannot injure them. A sudden, slight jerking and freeing of the tube will be sensed as the tip leaves the larynx and, following the same gentle curve as during insertion, it may now easily be removed from the mouth. At this point, however, the bronchoscopist should pause and carefully inspect the larynx, not only for possible trauma, but to assess active mobility of the cords, which should be returning spontaneously as the effects of anaesthesia diminish. It is at this stage, when general anaesthesia is used, and not during intubation, that possible recurrent laryngeal nerve paralysis may be discovered (Plate 8). While the tube is in this situation it is also convenient for the bronchoscopist to aspirate secretions from the pharynx (Fig. 16), although the anaesthetist may well prefer to do this himself. Finally, the lips, gums, teeth and tongue should be inspected for possible trauma, however carefully the procedure was carried out.

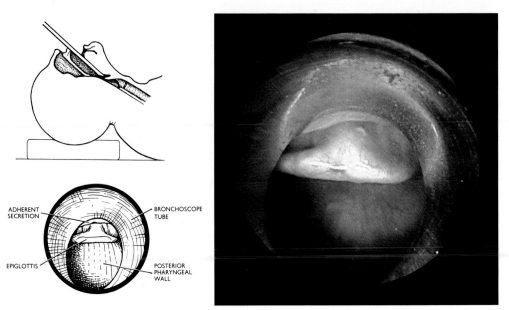

Plate 3

The epiglottis. The bronchoscope tip has followed the contour of the tongue towards its root and the epiglottis has been located and centred in the field of vision. Usually it is now a simple matter to slip the anteriorly placed tip of the tube posterior to the epiglottis and gently lift it forward. (Compare Fig. 8.)

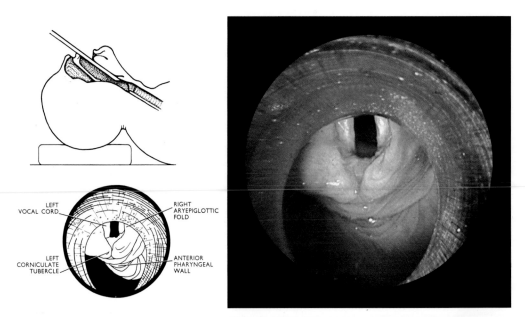

Plate 4

The entrance to the larynx. The tip of the bronchoscope, kept carefully in the midline, has now passed posterior to the free edge of the epiglottis which has been displaced gently but firmly forward. The posterior aspect of the laryngeal entrance has readily come into view. The posterior expansions of the aryepiglottic folds, and vocal cords beyond, are clearly seen. Failure to keep the bronchoscope in the midline at this stage leads to faulty positioning; usually in a pyriform fossa.

36

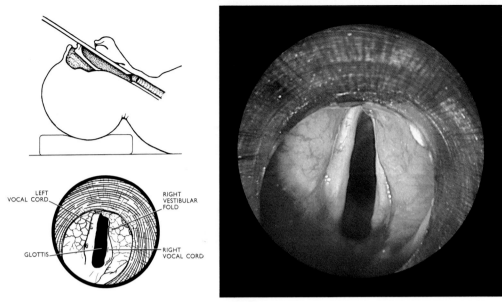

Plate 5

The larynx. Here the bronchoscope has been advanced a little further, after carefully aligning its axis with that of the glottis and trachea. The larynx has been entered by passing between the aryepiglottic folds and so revealing clearly the vestibular folds just proximal to the vocal cords. There is some asymmetry in this case; the right vestibular fold, protruding towards the midline, partially obscures the right vocal cord. (Compare Fig. 9.)

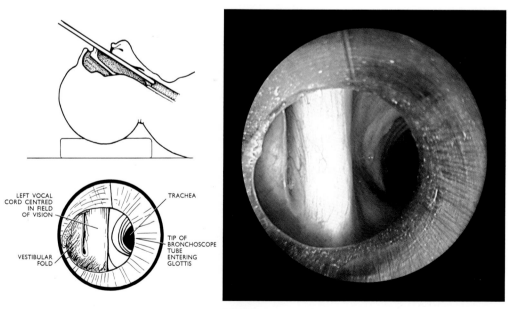

Plate 6

Negotiating the glottis. The tube has been rotated through 90° and the left vocal cord is centred in the field of vision: the bronchoscope tip is thus lying in the glottis. The instrument can now be insinuated gently through the glottis, with a slight twisting movement if necessary. Part of the left vestibular fold is seen on the left of the picture: on the right, tracheal cartilages can just be made out in the distance. (Compare Fig. 10.)

37

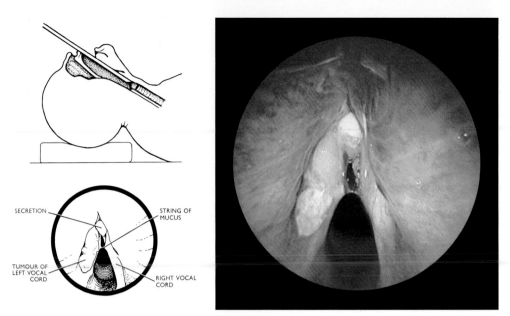

Plate 7

Carcinoma of larynx. There is an obvious tumour of the left vocal cord, possibly also involving the anterior commissure, which is obscured by mucopurulent secretion. This was a surprise finding during bronchoscopy done for suspicion of bronchial carcinoma on the left. The laryngeal symptoms were expected to be due to left vocal cord paresis. In fact the cords moved well. Biopsy: squamous-cell carcinoma.

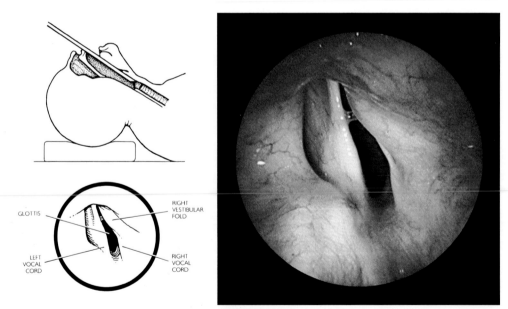

Plate 8

Vocal cord paralysis. The photograph was taken during early efforts at abduction as the patient was recovering from general anaesthesia. The right cord has moved laterally, almost to be hidden by the vestibular fold, but the left has remained in the neutral position. Vocal cord paralysis is much more commonly seen on the left because of the long intrathoracic course of the left recurrent laryngeal nerve rendering it liable to involvement in thoracic pathology. The condition will be missed if not looked for routinely at the *end* of any operation under general anaesthetia, when cord movement is returning. (Compare Plates 5, 99 & 163.)

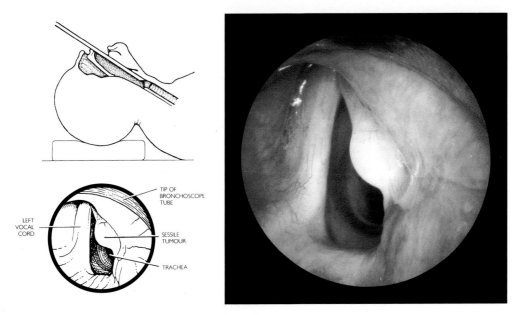

Plate 9

Benign tumour of right vocal cord. This was an incidental finding in a patient with carcinoma of the right intermediate bronchus. The cords moved normally and the patient had no laryngeal symptoms. Biopsy: benign polyp.

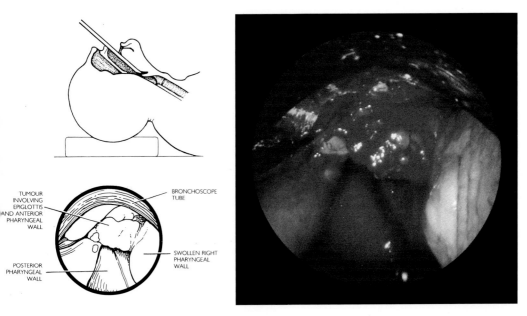

Plate 10

Pharyngeal carcinoma. Bronchoscopy was performed for repeated haemoptysis. Both the epiglottis and the right pharyngeal wall were grossly invaded and partially destroyed by carcinoma. This responded temporarily to radiotherapy.

CHAPTER 5

NORMALITY

Bronchial anatomy

Clinicians practising respiratory medicine obtain a sound knowledge of bronchial anatomy through constantly studying radiographic appearances of segmental pulmonary lesions. Nevertheless, a new and more complete appreciation of normal endobronchial morphology and its wide variations is essential if anatomical distortion and pathological changes are to be recognised bronchoscopically. If, at least, an outline of the normal endobronchial findings is studied before introducing the bronchoscope, this necessary knowledge will be gained more rapidly. The following chapter is designed to provide this background.

Branching is described sequentially, as encountered during passage of the bronchoscope, starting with the trachea, continuing down the right bronchial passages and finally returning to consider the left. A conventional diagram is provided for reference. In addition, key points in the bronchial tree are illustrated by endobronchial photographs and annotated drawings.* The exact position and viewing direction of the telescope objective lens is also indicated in each case. It is hoped that the combination of these methods of presentation will assist the student bronchoscopist to gain the knowledge of endobronchial anatomy necessary for further studies.

The prevailing pattern of anatomical normality is that given in the truncated outline diagram of the bronchial tree (Fig. 17). Only those branches whose orifices can usually be seen with rigid telescopes are depicted, but not infrequently more peripheral views can be obtained in individual cases (see also Fig. 18). The nomenclature widely accepted in the United Kingdom has been applied. This is similar to that used in the United States of America and thus there should be no confusion for American readers except in the case of the first, large, posteriorly directed branch of the lower bronchus on each side. American clinicians will know this as the *superior* bronchus, whereas an informal international committee, meeting in Britain in 1949, proposed that it should be called the *apical* bronchus. Both names can be criticised on the grounds of confusion: one with the apical branch of the upper bronchus and the other with the superior branch of the lingular. It is

---

*The word 'bronchus', which is required frequently in the annotations, is abbreviated to 'BR'. When the entry to a bronchus is seen only obliquely the word 'ORIFICE' usually replaces 'BR'.

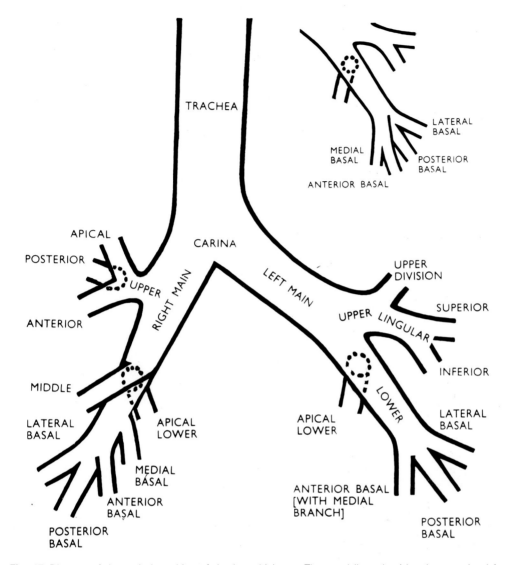

TRACHEA

LATERAL
BASAL

MEDIAL
BASAL

POSTERIOR
BASAL

ANTERIOR BASAL

APICAL

CARINA

UPPER
DIVISION

POSTERIOR

UPPER

RIGHT MAIN

LEFT MAIN

SUPERIOR

ANTERIOR

UPPER LINGULAR

MIDDLE

INFERIOR

LOWER

LATERAL
BASAL

APICAL
LOWER

APICAL
LOWER

LATERAL
BASAL

MEDIAL
BASAL

ANTERIOR
BASAL

ANTERIOR BASAL
[WITH MEDIAL
BRANCH]

POSTERIOR
BASAL

POSTERIOR
BASAL

Fig. 17 Diagram of the main branching of the bronchial tree. The word 'bronchus' has been omitted for simplification and to avoid repetition. The nomenclature is that widely used in the United Kingdom. (American readers see page 40). Adherence to a tripartite basal pattern on the left is not justified: a bipartite division with immediate subdivision (shown inset) is at least as common. Many other anatomical variations occur to give a wide range of normality.

sometimes called the *dorsal* bronchus, but the usual British practice is to call it the *apical lower* bronchus and this is adopted here.

The *trachea*, entered after passing the glottis, ends by dividing at the *carina* into the *right* and *left main* bronchi (Plate 11): the carina should be sharp and keel-like as its name implies (Plates 12, 13, 14 & 16). It usually appears nearly vertical to the bronchoscopist, but wide variation occurs and not infrequently it may lie at an angle of 45° from the vertical. Even at this level bronchial calibre can be seen to vary with respiration (Plates 13 & 14). Usually just beyond the carina, the right main bronchus (Plate 15) gives off the *right upper* bronchus which, in its turn and

41

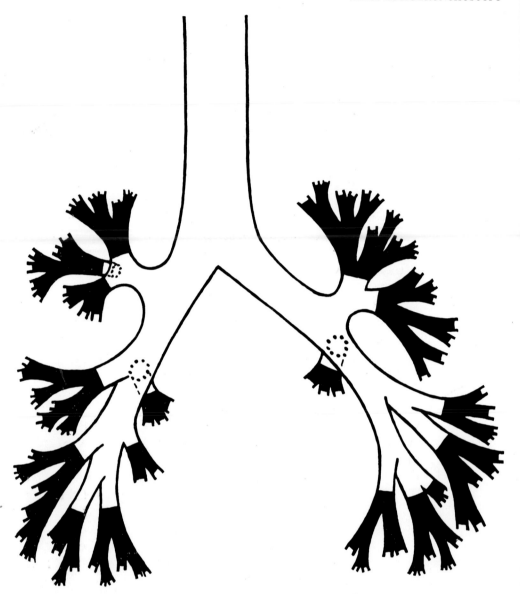

Fig. 18 The increased peripheral vision obtained by the fibrescope within the bronchial tree is here depicted in black. The illustration is not only diagrammatic but also can only approximate to any real situation. Individual anatomy varies considerably, not only in branching pattern but in the angulation of branches with their parent stems: both can have a marked effect on the depth of penetration obtained with the bronchofibrescope. Furthermore, rigid telescopes often provide greater penetration into the basal branches than depicted here.

immediately or very shortly, branches into three: the *apical*, *anterior* and *posterior* bronchi (Plate 17).

The *lower part of the right main* bronchus (i.e., that portion of the main bronchus that remains beyond the upper orifice and commonly called the *intermediate* bronchus) finally gives origin to the anteriorly directed *middle* bronchus, with its *lateral* and *medial* segmental branches, and so becomes the *right lower* bronchus (Plate 18). There may be a sudden narrowing at this point which results in a medial shelf;

this normal finding must not be confused with extrinsic pressure on the bronchus (Plates 16, 43 & 72). From the lower bronchus, a *right apical lower* bronchus immediately arises posteriorly (in fact, almost opposite the middle bronchus), and from a little lower, the *medial basal* bronchus arises medially (Plates 18 & 19). Finally the lower bronchus ends by dividing into the *right anterior, lateral* and *posterior basal* bronchi (Plates 18 & 19). These may either arise as three branches at the same level or the anterior basal bronchus arises first, the lower bronchus then terminating by dividing into posterior and lateral basal bronchi. Although these two methods of terminal branching of the lower bronchus are the commonest seen, there is great variability and it is not always possible to name the basal orifices with certainty (Plates 20, 21 & 22). However, in most cases, the placing of the orifices relative to each other, and the direction of the bronchial axes, make the position clear: the posterior basal bronchus is the most constant and is the direct continuation of the lower bronchus. Frequently, further, more distal divisions of the basal bronchi can be seen, even with rigid telescopes. The *right subapical* bronchus, supplying the separate subapical pulmonary segment, is more commonly present than not. It arises posteriorly, sometimes posteromedially or posterolaterally, at any position between the apical lower orifice and the final division into posterior and lateral basal bronchi (Plate 19). Otherwise it is an early branch of the posterior basal bronchus.

Returning to the carina, the bronchoscopist must now examine the left bronchial tree which presents fewer visible orifices than the right. The *left main* bronchus (Plate 23) makes more of an angle with the trachea, and descends further into the lung before dividing, than does the right main bronchus. It also curves a little laterally as it descends into the lung. The primary division, with a well-defined secondary carina, is into *left upper* bronchus and *left lower* bronchus (Plates 24 & 25). The left upper bronchus quickly divides into *upper division* and *lingular* bronchi (Plates 26, 27 & 28). The lingular bronchus is equivalent to the middle bronchus on the right and can often be seen, even with the forward-viewing rigid telescope, dividing into its *superior* and *inferior* branches (Plate 26).

There is great normal variation in the angle that the left upper bronchus makes with the main and lower bronchi, so that the excellence of the view, and the type of telescope needed to obtain it, vary accordingly. The axis of the secondary carina between the left upper and lower bronchi also varies considerably. Most commonly it lies obliquely between 8 o'clock and 2 o'clock on an imaginary clock face, but any position between the horizontal and vertical axes may be normal.

The left lower bronchus is longer than the right, and this, together with the somewhat higher origin of the posteriorly placed *left apical lower* bronchus (Plates 29 to 31 & 35), gives a greater distance between this branch and the *left basal* bronchi (Plates 25, 29 & 30). These basal branches frequently form a mirror image of those on the right (*anterior, lateral* and *posterior*) except that there is no separately arising medial basal bronchus (Plate 30). The left medial basal pulmonary segment is supplied by a branch of the large anterior basal bronchus when the lower bronchus ends in tripartition. An equally common finding, however, is a final termination of the lower bronchus in two main basal branches each of which almost immediately divides again. The more anterior branch gives origin to the *medial* and *anterior*

43

basal bronchi and the more posterior to the *posterior* and *lateral* basal bronchi. This pattern (Plate 33) provides a more obvious medial basal bronchus than does the triple division. Occasionally it is extremely difficult to classify the basal branching found into one of the two prevailing patterns and, without dissection, interpretation becomes a matter of opinion (Plates 31 & 32). A *subapical* bronchus is commonly present, but not so frequently as on the right (Plates 31 & 32).

Although this brief description outlines the more usual pattern of the major branches of the bronchial tree, there are many common variants, some of which are also illustrated here. The right upper bronchus frequently presents minor variations of its primary division or origin (Plate 16). The apical bronchus may arise separately, a varying distance from the common origin of the anterior and posterior branches (Plates 36 to 38): rarely, part of the upper lobe may receive its bronchial supply directly from the trachea (Plates 39 & 40). A true tracheal bronchus supplying an additional separate, small segment on the right is exceptionally rare. Sometimes one of the pulmonary segments of the upper lobe is supplied by two separate bronchi, instead of by one which subsequently divides: this gives the impression of four orifices instead of three at the origin of the right upper bronchus. Other cases may present a bifurcate pattern. Ultimate segmental distribution can only be determined by bronchography or dissection.

In some cases the left upper bronchus divides directly into three branches instead of two (Plate 163) and the subsequent variable peripheral distribution of these branches can be determined only by bronchography. The majority of such cases, however, represent a displacement of the anterior bronchus (usually a branch of the upper division) to a separate origin. In others the superior and inferior branches of the lingular bronchus may arise independently. In rare cases the upper division bronchus may arise directly from the main bronchus and more proximally than the lingular bronchus (Plate 47).

In the lungs of lower animals a series of large posterior branches arise from the stem bronchi. In man these are regularly represented by the apical lower and, commonly, by the subapical bronchi, having their origin in the lower bronchi. Additional posterior bronchial orifices, analogous with those in animals, are often seen, particularly on the right, sometimes proximal to the apical lower orifice, sometimes distal. The right apical lower pulmonary segment may itself have a split bronchial supply, one orifice being above, and the other below, the level of the middle bronchial orifice (Plate 43). Rarely the middle bronchus similarly may have a split origin (Plate 44).

Occasionally, a separately arising medial basal bronchus exists on the left and the anterior basal bronchus may be correspondingly small (Plate 34). Conversely the separate medial basal bronchus, usually found on the right, may be absent (Plates 22 & 124) and its territory is then supplied by branches from the anterior basal bronchus (and subapical if present). Rarely an additional *superior medial* bronchus may be present on the right, arising medially opposite, or nearly opposite, the upper bronchial orifice (Plates 41 & 42).

Although the commonest variations from the prevailing bronchial pattern have been mentioned, the bronchoscopist must be prepared to meet many other minor, and occasionally major, anomalies. One such is visceral transposition illustrated in

Plates 45 & 46. Anomalies of the bronchial cartilages, also, are not uncommon. They may lead to minor variations in cross-sectional shape of the trachea or bronchi (Plate 52), to cartilagenous spurs covered with normal mucosa (Plates 49 to 51), and sometimes to bizarre variations in bronchial morphology, obviously of developmental origin (Plate 48).

The bronchofibrescope provides a more peripheral view of the bronchial tree than that outlined in this brief anatomical survey. Whereas rigid telescopes can usually only visualise orifices at the third, and sometimes fourth, bronchial divisions, the most commonly used 5.0–5.5 mm diameter flexible instrument allows inspection routinely to the fourth division and usually to the fifth (Fig. 18). Anatomical variation at this level is great and beyond the scope of this book. For practical purposes, however, the position of a more peripheral lesion can be indicated sufficiently accurately by a combination of (a) careful wording and (b) placement on a diagram of the bronchial tree included on the bronchoscopy report form.

Bronchial wall structure

The supporting cartilages of the bronchial tree are often called 'rings', but this is a misnomer: usually, nowhere are they complete. The prevailing shape in the trachea and main bronchi is an incomplete circle, open posteriorly (Plates 11, 12, 15, 23 & 70); but considerable variation is encountered in the trachea where also they may be horseshoe, staple or arch-shaped. A posterior mobile membrane completes the tubular structure of this proximal part of the bronchial tree. In it is found a network of muscle fibres running in lattice fashion between the free ends of the incomplete cartilages. Lying internal to this muscle layer are long bundles of elastic fibres which frequently raise the mucosa into prominent longitudinal corrugations clearly visible to the bronchoscopist (Plates 12, 13, 15, 23, 37 & 50). The direction of these may help to locate the orifice of the right upper bronchus (Plate 50).

This membranous posterior wall takes part in the anatomical changes in the bronchial tree during respiration; it stretches during inspiration to assist in producing an almost circular bronchial lumen and protrudes forward slightly during expiration to give a more kidney-shaped cross-section (Plates 13 & 14). This change may be quite prominent on coughing or forced expiration, but if marked during normal respiratory excursions it is clearly abnormal (Plates 69 to 76). Examinations made on relaxed patients under general anaesthesia mask these changes, particularly the degree of forward displacement on expiration. An imitation of inspiratory expansion of the lumen can, however, be reproduced by using the Sanders ventilator to raise the intrabronchial pressure (Plates 13, 14, 69 & 70). A small, but prominent, forward protrusion of the posterior tracheal wall just beyond the glottis is a common, normal finding.

More peripherally in the main and lobar bronchi the elements of their walls become progressively rearranged. The cartilages break up into irregular plates scattered in random fashion around the walls to form their outer, rigid support. The posterior membranous wall becomes steadily narrower and finally disappears as the muscular and elastic elements become continuous round the circumference of the bronchial lumen. The mucosa is thus raised from the cartilages by the interposing muscle and by the longitudinal elastic bundles, which frequently can be seen to corrugate the mucosa surrounding the whole lumen instead of only on the posterior wall (Plate 77). This transformation is usually complete at the lobar to segmental bronchial level and provides a mobile, musculoelastic lining to a more rigid outer tube: any changes involving muscle and elastic tissue will now produce circumferential effects instead of in the posterior wall only. The mucosa, no longer firmly adherent to cartilage, can readily collapse intraluminally, away from the bronchial wall, when muscular contraction takes place. Since such contraction both constricts and shortens the bronchi at this level and the longitudinal elastic bundles shorten and thicken at the same time, mucosal corrugation can be very prominent when bronchial muscle contracts. When mucosal swelling is also present, as in some cases of chronic bronchitis, the effect is exaggerated still further (Ch. 6).

Bronchial mucosa

The colour of the bronchial mucosa can vary greatly with the intensity and type of lighting used in the bronchoscope: each operator must familiarise himself with normality under his own, standardised conditions. Furthermore, the limitations of colour photography and printing must constantly be borne in mind when studying the photographs in this chapter and Chapter 6. Only an approximation to natural colour has been achieved.

The mucosa throughout the bronchial tree is normally of a pale pink or flesh tint (Plates 11, 15, 39 & 101), and often fine vessels can just be seen creating a delicate tracery, particularly around the carina and in the main bronchi. These vessels are most prominent in the intercartilagenous grooves and thin out over the cartilages themselves (Plates 23 & 101). In the lighting conditions used for bronchoscopy, the moist mucosal surface glistens noticeably. Highlights are particularly frequent and are reflected from portions of mucosa offering a flat surface at right angles to the lighting source—such as that lying on carinae, prominent cartilages, or protuberances into bronchi (Plates 12, 17, 26 & 50). Normal mucosa and submucosa form a thin membrane closely following all contours of the tracheal and bronchial walls, thus clearly revealing the presence or absence of supporting cartilage, mucous duct orifices or any small changes in the walls (Plates 17, 50, 58 & 181).

The normal mucosa blushes readily and rapidly on slight trauma, as can clearly be demonstrated by passing the bronchoscope distally until it fits snugly in the intubated bronchus: the blanching created by this slight pressure is rapidly followed by reactive hyperaemia sufficient to produce a marked change in the depth of colour, or even ecchymosis (Plates 12 & 33). Use of a sucker tube can also readily produce hyperaemia (Plates 183 & 184), ecchymosis or even minor bleeding (Plate 189). Great gentleness is thus at a premium if a true appreciation of the mucosal state is to be obtained.

A very thin surface layer of mucus, in which the cilia beat, gives the mucosa its characteristic shine (Plate 26). Being part of the normal cleansing mechanism of the bronchial tree, it is acceptable in normality but only in small quantity, often as occasional local collections (Plate 15). It may be swept into larger collections by the leading edge of the bronchoscope, thus giving a false impression of its quantity. Such amounts do not denote excessive secretion, but, once a sucker is required, abnormal mucus production is occurring. Even in normal subjects, mucous duct orifices occasionally can be seen lying in the mucosa where the cartilages make an angle with the posterior membranous bronchial wall: they appear as small pin-sized pits and are particularly likely to be seen on the posteromedial aspect of both main bronchi just beyond the carina and on the inferior walls of both upper bronchi. The dilated orifices seen in chronic bronchitis are discussed in Chapter 6.

In the elderly a common and normal age change is a degree of submucosal atrophy. The intercartilagenous grooves in the larger bronchial passages deepen with this atrophy, throwing the cartilages and carinae into sharper relief (Plate 12).

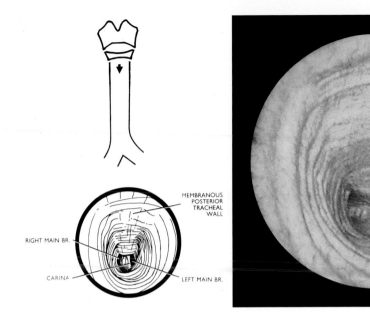

MEMBRANOUS
POSTERIOR
TRACHEAL
WALL

RIGHT MAIN BR.

CARINA

LEFT MAIN BR.

Plate 11

Normal trachea. The contours of the cartilages are well seen covered by pale, healthy mucosa, containing a network of fine vessels. Less light is reflected from the intercartilagenous grooves and from the flat posterior membranous wall: hence these areas are normally darker and redder in colour. Longitudinal mucosal corrugations on the posterior membranous wall are not always prominent and here are suggested only faintly. The carina and orifices of right and left main bronchi can be seen in the distance.

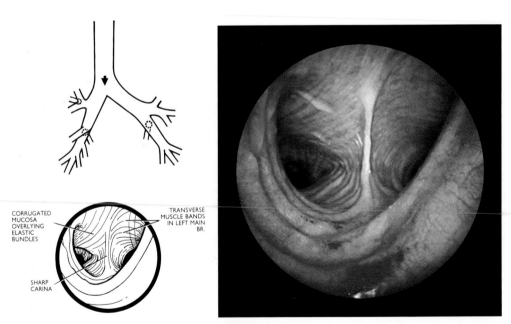

CORRUGATED
MUCOSA
OVERLYING
ELASTIC
BUNDLES

TRANSVERSE
MUSCLE BANDS
IN LEFT MAIN
BR.

SHARP
CARINA

Plate 12

Normal carina. The carinal edge in this case is extremely sharp. The submucosa is thin, showing some senile atrophy, and the mucosa is drawn tightly over the carina and cartilages. The posterior longitudinal mucosal corrugations outlining the elastic bundles, can be seen clearly but are not prominent. The mucosa is a little reddened and there is an increase in secretion due to mild bronchitis. The minor ecchymosis, seen on the anterior tracheal wall in the lower part of the picture, is due to slight pressure from the bronchoscope tube.

48

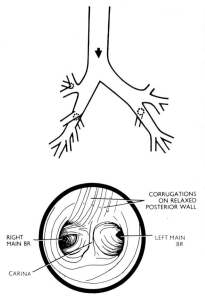

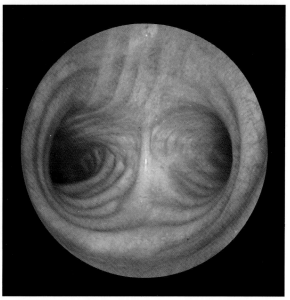

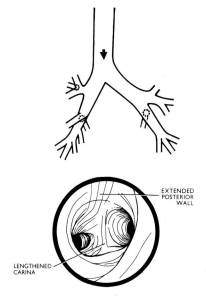

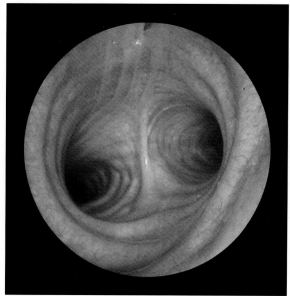

Plates 13 & 14

Normal carina. Changes with quiet respiration. The keel-like carinal edge is sharp and prominent as its name implies. The bronchial cartilage outlines are clearly seen beyond the carina, more so in the straighter right main bronchus, which is normally visible to a greater depth than the left. Posterior longitudinal mucosal corrugations are well seen, particularly in the lower trachea and the right main bronchus. The forward protrusion of the posterior walls during the expiratory phase, or during relaxation under general anaesthesia, is slight in normal subjects (Plate 13). It is rapidly abolished by raising the intrabronchial pressure, either by inspiration or ventilation (Plate 14); the lumina became more circular in outline and the transverse muscle bands may be seen more readily, in this case particularly in the left main bronchus. (Compare Plates 69 to 74, 97, 98 and 102.)

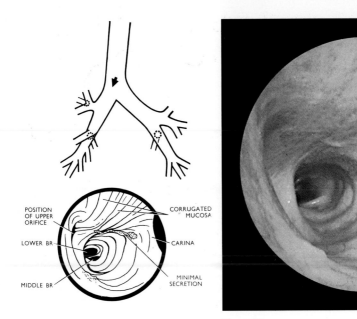

Plate 15

Normal right main bronchus. The cartilage outlines are well seen through the mucosa as far as the final division into middle and lower bronchi. The inferior lip of the upper bronchial orifice stands out well, making the orifice itself easy to locate. The longitudinal mucosal corrugations on the posterior wall are not unduly prominent and the carina is sharp. The minimal secretion, seen on the posterior wall, has been swept into a transverse string by the bronchoscope tube.

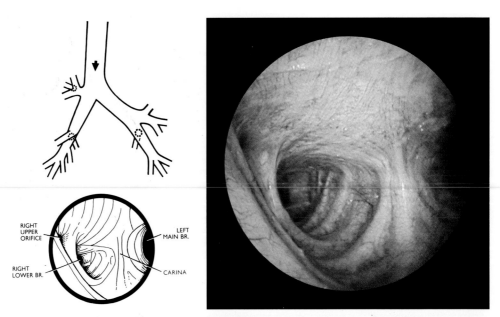

Plate 16

Main bifurcation. High origin of right upper bronchus. The carina is normally sharp and the cartilages are well seen. The lower lip of the right upper orifice is opposite the carinal edge and thus the upper bronchus is arising just within the trachea. (Compare Plate 15.) Variations in the position of this bronchus are common. In the distance can be seen a medial shelf at the level of the bifurcation of the intermediate bronchus. This sudden narrowing of the lumen must not be mistaken for pathological distortion. (Compare Plates 42, 43 & 72).

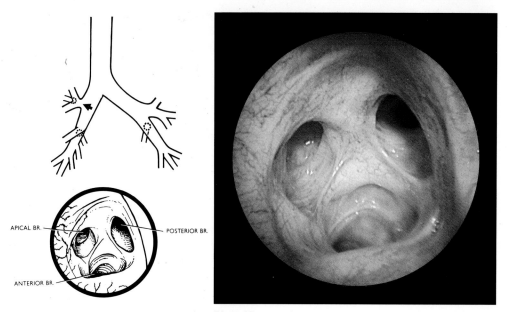

Plate 17

Normal right upper bronchial orifice. Lateral-viewing telescope. The normal tripartite primary division of the upper bronchus into anterior, posterior and apical branches is well seen here, occurring immediately after its origin. It is for the further investigation of these branches, and those of the left upper bronchus, that the fibrescope is particularly valuable. The mucosa is healthy and shows the normal delicate tracery of mucosal vessels.

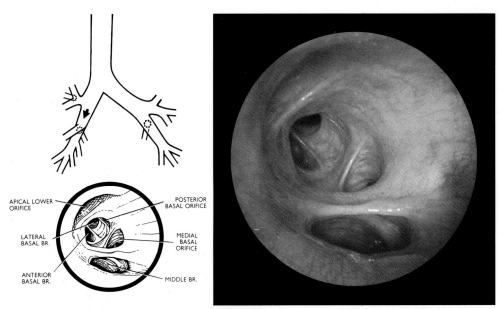

Plate 18

Normal termination of right main (intermediate) bronchus. The large middle bronchial orifice, semilunar in shape, lies anteriorly. A prominent secondary carina separates it from the lower bronchus which immediately gives origin to the posteriorly placed apical lower bronchus. This orifice (whether left or right) usually can only be inspected with a lateral-viewing telescope or fibrescope. (See Plate 35.) The orifice of the medial basal bronchus, also often semilunar in outline, is placed distal to the apical lower orifice and is clearly seen on the medial wall of the lower bronchus before its final branching into the three basal bronchi. In this case, as is common, the posterior basal orifice cannot be identified clearly without further advancing the telescope.

51

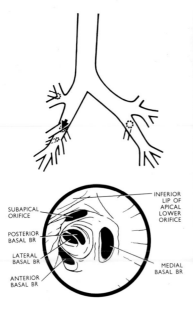

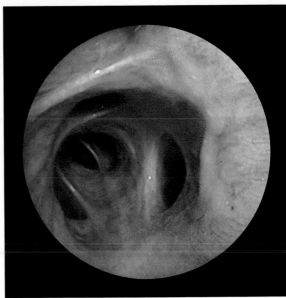

Plate 19

Normal branching of right lower bronchus. The inferior margin of the apical lower bronchus is just visible at the periphery. Immediately distal to this, on the posterior wall, is seen the orifice of the subapical bronchus, arising in this case proximal to the medial basal bronchus. The pattern of the remaining basal branching is one very commonly seen: a large medial basal branch (to the right of centre), an anterior branch (to the far left) and the lower bronchus finally terminating (in the distance) by dividing into lateral and posterior basal bronchi.

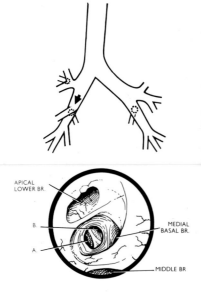

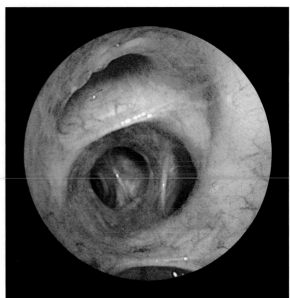

Plate 20

Normal variation of right lower branching. The posterior margin of the middle bronchial orifice is just visible at the bottom of the picture. At the top is the large apical lower orifice. Beyond this is seen a prominent medial basal orifice and the lower bronchus terminates in a bipartite division (A & B), instead of the usual tripartite into anterior, lateral and posterior basal bronchi. The distribution of these two branches could only be determined by bronchography or dissection.

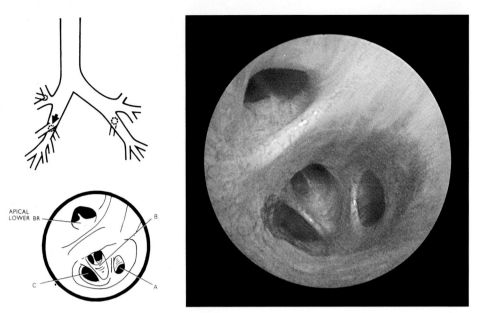

Plate 21

Normal variation of right lower branching. The apical lower bronchus passes obliquely inferoposteriorly instead of in the more usual posterior direction. A prominent secondary carina is thus present and a partial view of the primary branching of this bronchus can be obtained with the forward-viewing telescope. The exact ditribution of the final basal branching could only be ascertained by bronchography for there are three orifices at the same level (here named A, B and C), the most posterior (B) dividing rapidly. The most likely designation is: A = medial basal, B = posterior and lateral basals, C = anterior basal.

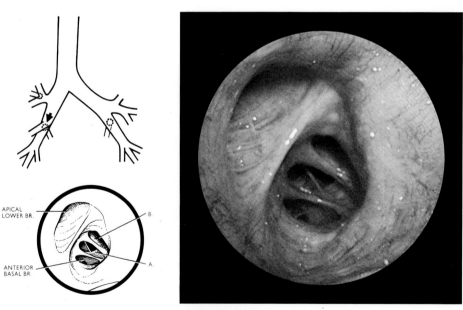

Plate 22

Normal variation of right lower branching. The apical lower bronchus is larger than usual and passes laterally and slightly downwards. The basal branching is unusual in that there is no obviously separate medial basal bronchus: only three orifices are seen at the same level. It is clear that the most anteriorly placed branch is the anterior basal bronchus but there are two possible designations for orifices A and B: (1) A = common origin of lateral and posterior basal bronchi, B = displaced medial basal bronchus; (2) A = lateral basal bronchus, B = posterior basal bronchus. In the latter case the territory normally supplied by a separate medial basal bronchus would probably receive branches from the unusually large apical lower bronchus and possibly from the anterior and posterior basal bronchi.

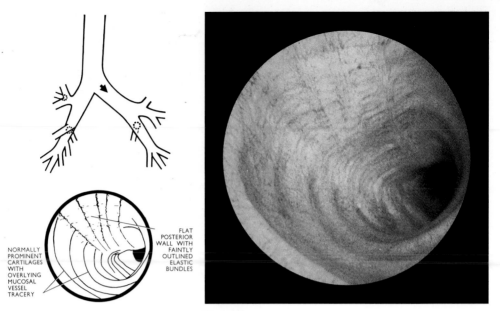

NORMALLY PROMINENT CARTILAGES WITH OVERLYING MUCOSAL VESSEL TRACERY

FLAT POSTERIOR WALL WITH FAINTLY OUTLINED ELASTIC BUNDLES

Plate 23

Normal left main bronchus. The normal gentle lateral curve, well seen here, explains the necessity for progressive movement of the head to the right when passing a rigid tube down the left main bronchus. It also prevents clear visualisation of the final division into upper and lower bronchi from this level. Prominent bronchial cartilages, faintly visible mucosal corrugations on the posterior membranous wall and the delicate vessel tracery in the mucosa are all well seen.

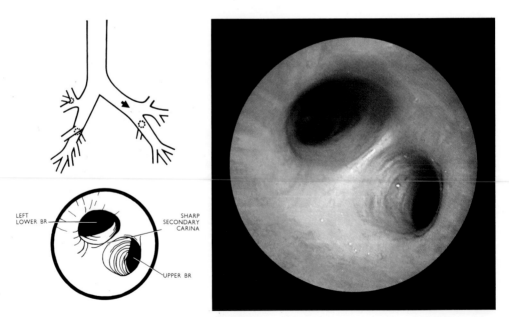

LEFT LOWER BR

SHARP SECONDARY CARINA

UPPER BR

Plate 24

Normal division of left main bronchus. The secondary carina is sharp. The upper bronchus makes an angle of about 60° with the main bronchus and thus only its orifice can be seen: a lateral or oblique-viewing telescope, or, even better, the fibrescope, would be needed to see its divisions. The lower bronchus is almost a direct continuation of the main bronchus and its basal divisions can be seen very dimly in the distance.

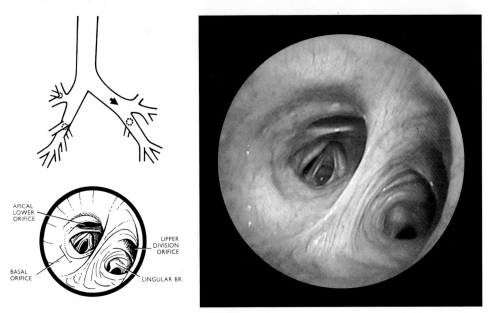

APICAL
LOWER
ORIFICE

UPPER
DIVISION
ORIFICE

BASAL
ORIFICE

LINGULAR BR.

Plate 25

Normal division of left main bronchus. In this instance, the upper bronchus makes a very acute angle with the common axis of the main and lower bronchi; this is one end of the range of normal possibilities of which a right-angled origin is the other. In consequence, it is possible, from the same vantage point, to see well into both upper and lower bronchi. The secondary carina is knife sharp, and set, as usual, at an oblique angle to the antero-posterior axis.

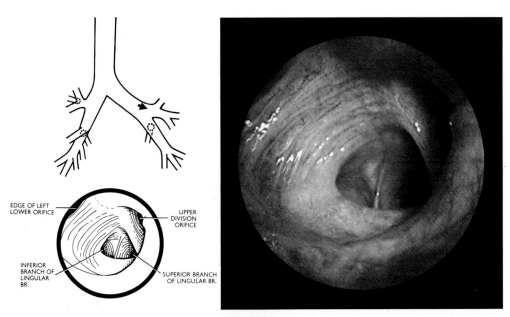

EDGE OF LEFT
LOWER ORIFICE

UPPER
DIVISION
ORIFICE

INFERIOR
BRANCH OF
LINGULAR
BR.

SUPERIOR BRANCH
OF LINGULAR BR.

Plate 26

Normal left upper bronchus. Frequently, as in this case, it is possible to see directly into the upper bronchus with the forward viewing rigid telescope. The edge of the prominent secondary carina between upper and lower bronchi is just seen at the picture periphery. The bifurcation of the lingular bronchus into its superior and inferior branches is clearly seen. An oblique view only is obtained of the upper division orifice. The fibre-scope is of particular value for further investigation of these branches.

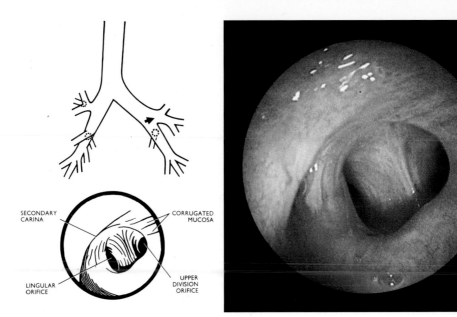

Plate 27

Normal left upper bronchus. Lateral-viewing telescope. The lateral-viewing instrument or the fibrescope is commonly necessary to see the left upper bronchus and its primary division. Part of the secondary carina between upper and lower bronchi is seen on the left of the picture. It is casting a deep shadow on the inferior, curved wall of the upper bronchus. This frequently occurs and should not be mistaken for another orifice. The bronchus divides shortly after its origin and here, as is often the case, the angle between upper division and lingular bronchi is such that their orifices are only partly visualised with rigid telescopes. (Compare Plate 28.)

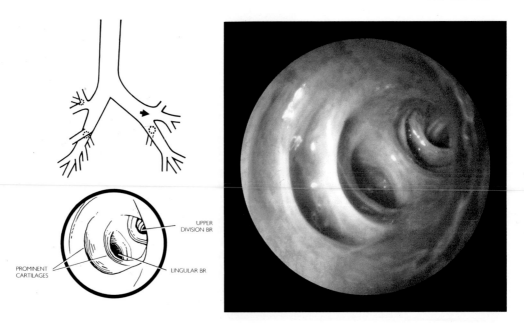

Plate 28

Normal left upper bronchus. Oblique-viewing telescope. The findings are similar to those in Plate 27. The lingular and upper division orifices are well seen. In addition heavy shadows are cast on the inferior wall of the upper bronchus, suggesting possible additional orifices. In fact these are caused by the rather prominent cartilages, so common in this area.

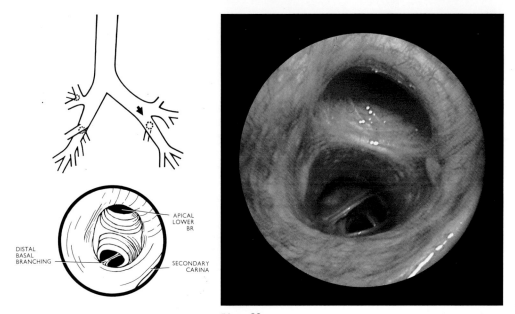

Plate 29

Normal left lower bronchus. The secondary carina between upper and lower bronchi is just visible at the picture periphery. The large, apical lower bronchial orifice is well seen and at least two major basal bronchi can be made out in the distance. As is frequently the case, the details of this division cannot be determined from this level. Some mucosal hyperaemia is present but no marked swelling or excess secretion.

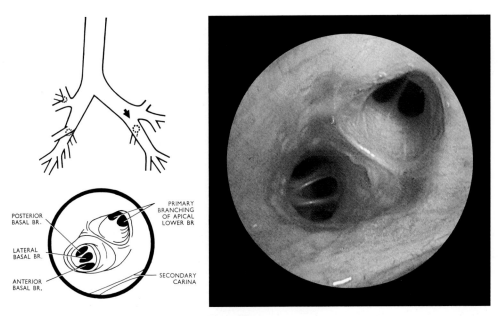

Plate 30

Normal variation of left lower branching. Part of the secondary carina separating upper and lower bronchi is at the periphery of the picture. Another prominent secondary carina separates the lower bronchus from its large apical lower branch, which passes obliquely downwards and backwards to allow a view of its primary division with the forward-viewing telescope. The final lower bronchial branching, seen in the distance, is of a common normal pattern: tripartite division into anterior, lateral and posterior basal bronchi.

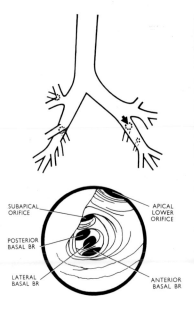
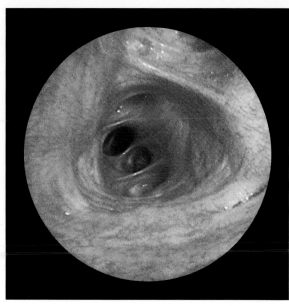

SUBAPICAL
ORIFICE

APICAL
LOWER
ORIFICE

POSTERIOR
BASAL BR

LATERAL
BASAL BR

ANTERIOR
BASAL BR

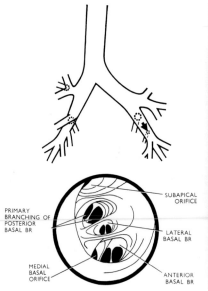
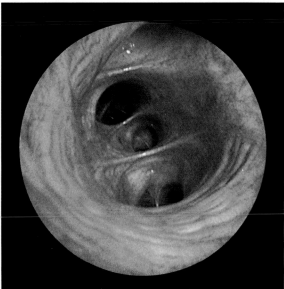

PRIMARY
BRANCHING OF
POSTERIOR
BASAL BR

SUBAPICAL
ORIFICE

LATERAL
BASAL BR

MEDIAL
BASAL
ORIFICE

ANTERIOR
BASAL BR

Plates 31 & 32

Normal variant of the left lower branching. Subapical bronchus present. In Plate 31, part of the apical lower orifice is at the picture periphery. The final division, apparently into three basal bronchi, is seen in the distance. Between the apical lower orifice and the basal bronchi lies the orifice of an additional subapical bronchus, commonly seen on the left, but not so frequently as on the right. In Plate 32 the telescope has been advanced further so that the subapical orifice is now only partially seen and the pattern of basal branching can be studied more clearly. The large anterior basal bronchus arises just before the smaller posterior and lateral basal bronchi and immediately supplies, via a medial branch, the medial basal pulmonary segment. This variant lies between the more obvious tripartite and bipartite patterns commonly seen.

58

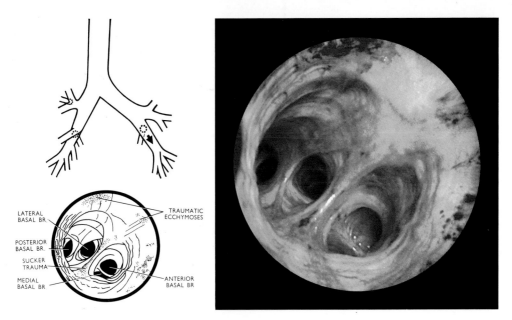

Plate 33

Normal left basal branching. The pattern is a clear example of bipartite division of the lower bronchus. These two branches provide common origins for (a) the anterior and medial, and (b) the lateral and posterior, basal bronchi. Round the bronchial circumference, at the periphery of the photograph, are numerous ecchymoses. These have been produced by pressure from the bronchoscope tube, introduced to its limit to allow the best possible view. The mucosa is very delicate and only slight pressure will often produce this effect. The degree of damage is insignificant: its importance lies in possible confusion with non-iatrogenic pathology. (Compare Plates 170, 189 & 225.)

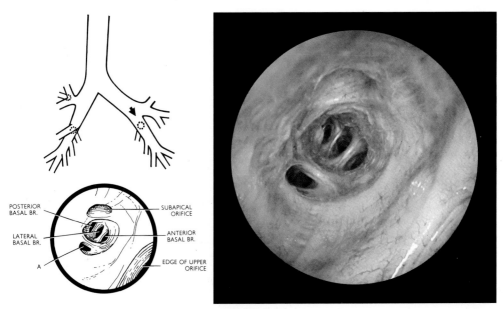

Plate 34

Variation of left lower branching. The secondary carina between upper and lower bronchi is at the right lower periphery of the picture: the subapical orifice at the top. The distal basal branching is of one common pattern, the three bronchi arising at the same level. An additional orifice (A) is present in the anterior wall of the lower bronchus and this probably supplies the medial basal pulmonary segment, more usually supplied from the anterior basal bronchus. (Compare Plates 32 & 177.)

59

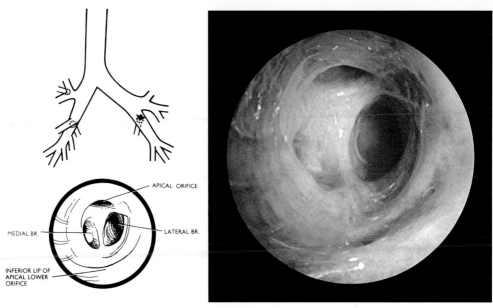

Plate 35

Normal left apical lower bronchus. Lateral-viewing telescope. Although occasionally visualised with a forward-viewing telescope, if of very oblique origin, the apical lower bronchus usually can only be seen clearly with an oblique telescope, the lateral-viewing instrument turned to view posteriorly, or with the fibrescope. The normal pattern of branching is that shown here; an apical branch arising first and then termination by division into medial and lateral branches.

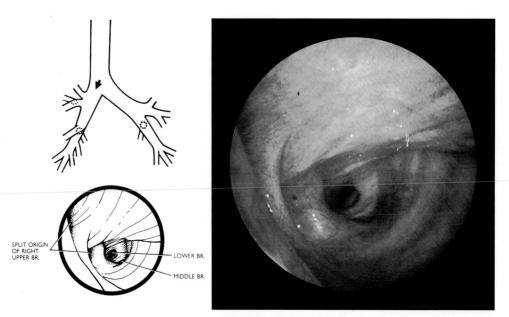

Plate 36

Double origin of right upper bronchus. Here the separation of the apical bronchus from the anterior and posterior bronchi has gone a stage further than illustrated in Plates 37 & 38: the apical branch has a completely separate origin. Although it is likely that this is the interpretation of the findings, one cannot be certain without bronchography or dissection. (Compare also Plate 39.) There was some bronchitis present in this patient, associated with mucosal flaccidity: hence the forward displacement of the posterior wall.

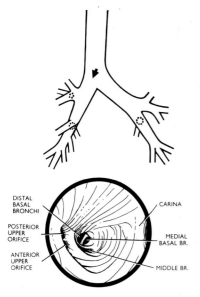

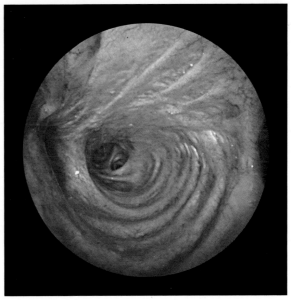

DISTAL BASAL BRONCHI — CARINA

POSTERIOR UPPER ORIFICE

ANTERIOR UPPER ORIFICE

MEDIAL BASAL BR.

MIDDLE BR.

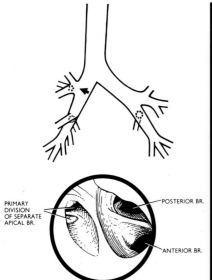

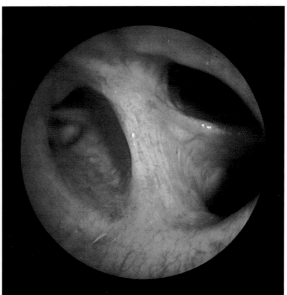

PRIMARY DIVISION OF SEPARATE APICAL BR.

POSTERIOR BR.

ANTERIOR BR.

Plates 37 & 38

Normal variant of right upper orifice. Plate 37 illustrates a normal right main bronchus with the carina to the far right and the division into middle and lower bronchi in the distance. The posterior longitudinal corrugations are well seen, those on the left leading to the unusually large right upper orifice, its lower lip more prominent than usual. Plate 38 is a view with the lateral-viewing telescope and shows the reason for the large opening: the apical bronchus is well separated from the other two. Its bifurcation can be seen in the distance. Variations on this theme are commonly found.

61

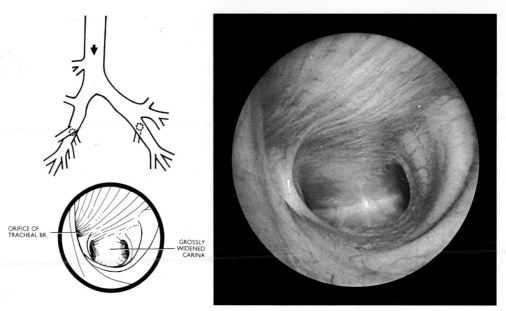

Plate 39

Tracheal bronchus. This is clearly seen as a large additional bronchus passing laterally from the right wall of the trachea. In this case it represents a developmental variation of the bronchial supply to the right upper lobe. A small, single orifice was present in the usual position for the right upper bronchus and bronchography revealed that only the posterior pulmonary segment was supplied by this bronchus: the tracheal bronchus led to both the anterior and apical segments. An additional feature of this case is the presence of a large, benign tumour in the mediastinum which has greatly widened the carina. The overlying mucosa remains normal, as is usual with benign tumours. (Compare Plate 40.)

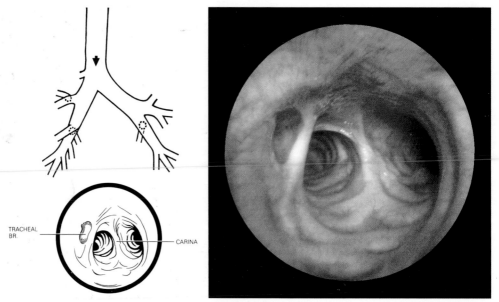

Plate 40

Tracheal bronchus. In this case, the additional orifice is seen more distally in the trachea than in Plate 39. It represents displacement of only the apical branch of the right upper bronchus: both anterior and posterior branches were found in their usual positions. The mucosa is normal and there is only minimal secretion on the posterior wall of the right main branchus.

62

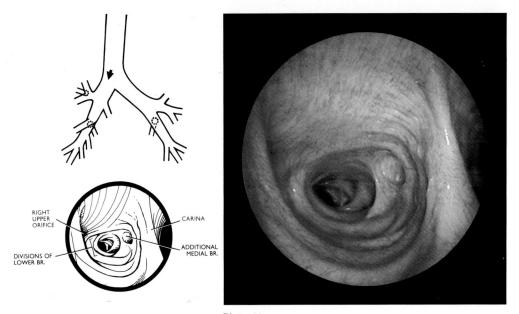

Plate 41

Additional superior medial branch of right main bronchus. The carina is well seen on the right; the division of the intermediate bronchus in the distance. The posterior corrugations are faintly visible, leading to the upper bronchus as usual. The additional bronchus can be seen cleary to the right of the picture centre, arising from the medial wall and passing downwards and medially. This is a rare finding. (Compare Plate 42.)

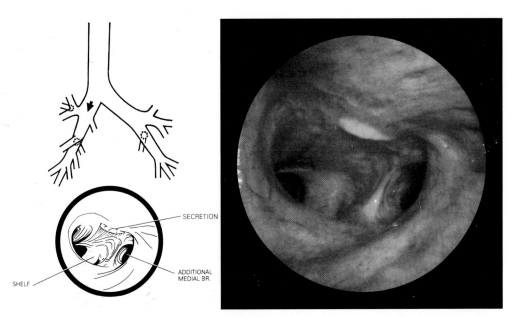

Plate 42

Additional superior medial branch of right main bronchus. In this case the additional bronchus is much larger than in Plate 41 and is clearly seen right of centre. There is slight mucosal swelling and excess secretion consistant with mild chronic bronchitis. A medial shelf is seen in the distance at the point of division of the intermediate bronchus. (Compare Plates 16, 41, 43 & 72.)

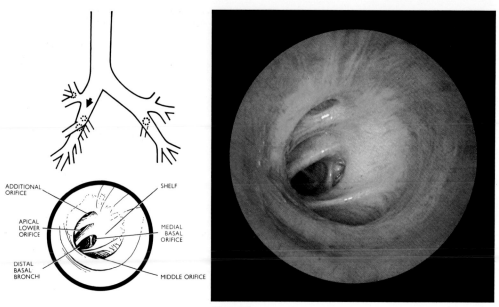

Plate 43

Double origin of apical lower bronchus. On the posterior wall and proximal to the level of the middle bronchus, is an additional orifice. This is only slightly smaller than that seen more distally in the usual place for the apical lower bronchus. This is the common pattern for a double origin, apical lower bronchus: one orifice proximal and one distal to the middle orifice. A medial shelf is also present. (Compare Plates 16, 42 & 72.)

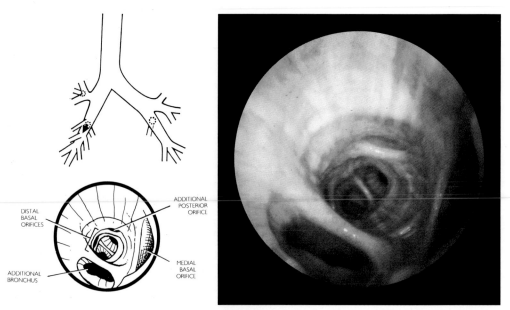

Plate 44

Double origin of middle bronchus. The photograph is taken just beyond the termination of the intermediate bronchus so that the smaller, more proximal, origin of the middle bronchus and the apical lower bronchus are not seen. A large additional orifice is seen anteriorly, positioned proximal to the normally-patterned orifices of the medial basal bronchus and more distal basal bronchi. There is also a small distally placed subapical bronchus present; a common finding. The small size of the normally-positioned middle orifice suggests that the large additional bronchus supplies a major part of the middle lobe.

64

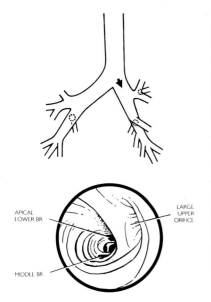

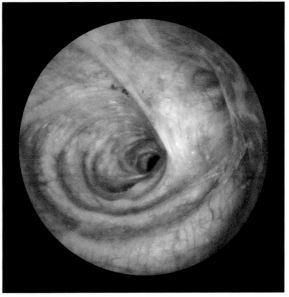

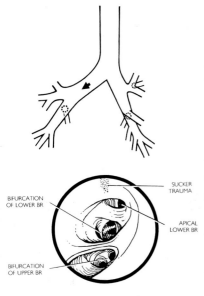

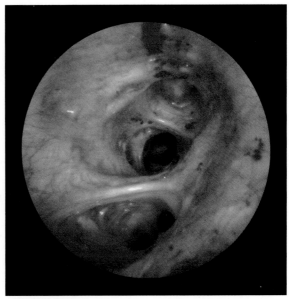

Plates 45 and 46

Visceral transposition. The bronchial pattern on each side is a mirror image of that normally found on the other. Plate 45 shows clearly the left main bronchus with the upper bronchial orifice to the right and the division into the middle and lower bronchi in the distance. The division of the right main bronchus (Plate 46) is well illustrated, showing the orifices to upper, apical lower and basal bronchi. This patient, with transposed viscera, suffered from nasal sinusitis and basal bronchiectasis (Kartagener's Syndrome). The profuse purulent secretion present on both sides was aspirated before photography: hence the minor sucker trauma seen in both plates.

65

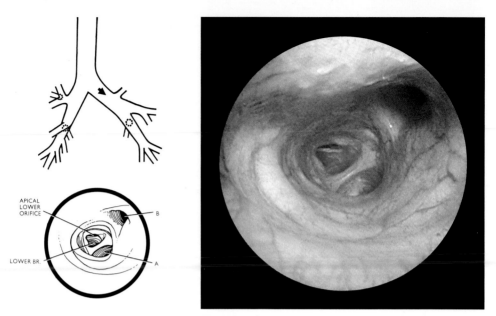

Plate 47

Anomalous branching of the left main bronchus. An apparently normal branching into upper and lower bronchi is seen in the distance: the apical lower orifice is found in its usual posterior position. The territory supplied by the apparent upper bronchus (A) is, however, in doubt because of the presence of an additional orifice (B) located postero-laterally and more proximally in the main bronchus. Presumably this anomalous branch supplies all, or part, of the territory normally supplied by the upper division of the upper bronchus: a situation analogous to proximal displacement of the apical bronchus on the right. Bronchography or dissection would be required to establish the true position.

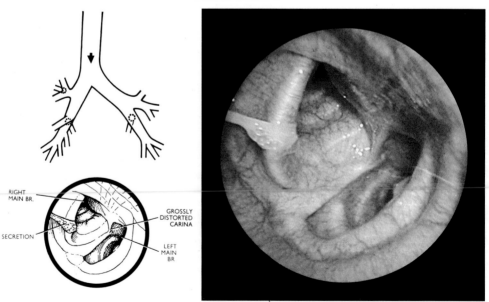

Plate 48

Anomalous main bifurcation. The right and left main bronchial orifices are not strictly side by side as is usual: the left is more anteriorly placed than the right. The angulation to the right of the anterior part of the carina gives an oval contour to the left main orifice and is associated with a clockwise twist of the right main bronchus. The membranous portion of the right main bronchus becomes more medial than posterior, the upper orifice more posterior than lateral. A curl of secretion is issuing from the right main bronchus. Minor degrees of this anomaly are quite common—the carina being twisted to left or right. (Compare Plates 93 & 198.)

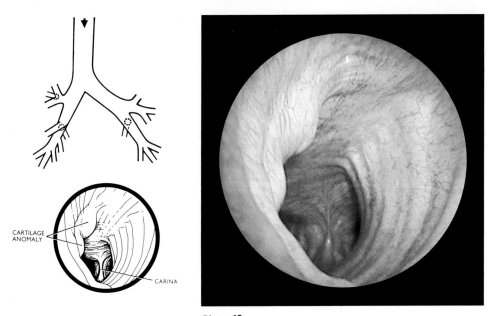

Plate 49

Cartilagenous anomaly. Trachea. On the lateral wall of the mid trachea is seen a bilobed distortion of one of the cartilages. The overlying mucosa is normal in colour and smooth, with a delicate vessel tracery visible. This was a local phenomenon; the sharp carina and other, normal, cartilages are well seen in the distance.

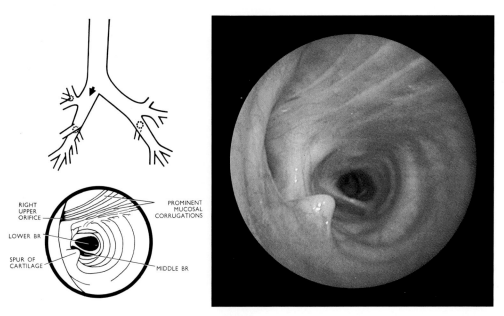

Plate 50

Cartilagenous anomaly. Right main bronchus. The patient was mildly bronchitic: the prominent posterior corrugations clearly delineate the elastic bundles and indicate the position of the upper orifice. Placed antero-laterally, and arising from a bronchial cartilage at the level of the upper orifice, is a cartilagenous spur with pale overlying mucosa. Biopsy revealed normal cartilage. (Compare Plate 176.)

67

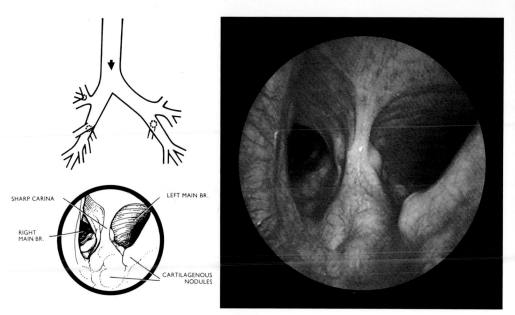

Plate 51

Cartilagenous anomaly. Main bifurcation. There is generalised reddening of the mucosa with a marked increase in vascularity due to chronic bronchitis. The anterior carina and the proximal cartilages of the main bronchi are studded with nodules. There was a suspicion that these might be metastatic deposits of carcinoma from a known tumour in the left lower bronchus, but the sharp carina was against this possibility. Negative biopsies and identical bronchoscopic findings two years later confirmed the diagnosis. (Compare Plates 137 & 138.)

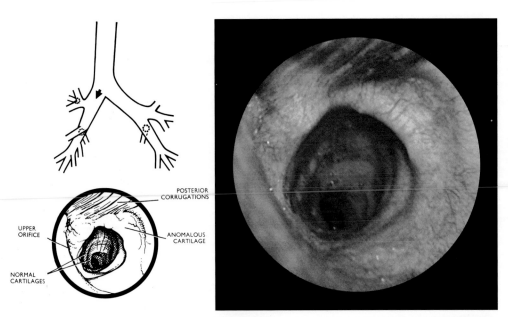

Plate 52

Cartilagenous anomaly. Right main bronchus. There is generalised reddening of the mucosa, due to chronic bronchitis, with mucopurulent secretion present, seen distally in the centre of the picture. The membranous posterior wall of the main bronchus is interrupted, just distal to the upper orifice, by a prominent cartilage which has formed a complete ring at this point. This could easily be confused with tumour spreading in the bronchial wall. (Compare Plate 147.)

CHAPTER 6

INFLAMMATORY AND
ASSOCIATED CHANGES

There are few ways in which the bronchial mucosa and submucosa can react to irritation or infection but, since the mucosa forms a thin surface membrane open to inspection over a wide area, these changes can be seen readily through the bronchoscope. Increased vascularity, reddening, swelling, irregularity and increased mucus secretion are most commonly seen. In the presence of microbial infection, pus formation and, occasionally, ulceration are added. Long-standing chronic conditions may lead to the formation of granulation tissue; healing processes can produce contractive scarring. Inflammatory changes may be generalised (usually chronic bronchitis) or localised (for example round a foreign body), acute (for example associated with segmental pneumonia) or chronic (for example tuberculosis), but the different changes vary considerably in degree in individual patients with the same condition. Conversely, since the mucosa can only react in the limited ways stated above, different pathological conditions can produce remarkably similar pictures. It is thus often difficult, or indeed sometimes impossible, to state a cause for the nonspecific inflammatory changes found.

Reddening and increased vascularity

A distinct reddening of the normally pale pink, or peach-coloured, bronchial mucosa is the most constant sign of inflammatory change. Patients that come to bronchoscopy are so commonly bronchitic that one must guard against accepting a deep red colouration as the normal: it can be a pleasant reminder of true normality to find pale mucosa when examining a young, healthy, nonsmoking adult.

The reddening may consist of simple engorgement of the larger mucosal vessels (making them more prominent and apparently much more numerous than usual), a more generalised bright pink, varying shades of red or a deeper 'raw beef' appearance. Colour changes are so subtle and the difficulties of accurate photographic recording and printing are so great, that again, the reader must be reminded that only an approximation to the actual colouring can be claimed here. Student bronchoscopists can only be guided by the ensuing plates (53 to 55, 59 & 61): more confident interpretation of findings will follow experience with their own apparatus. Numerous other examples of inflammatory reddening and vascularity occur in this book and comparison can be made, for instance, with Plates 51, 129, 130, 224 & 225.

Swelling

Swelling of the bronchial mucosa is also a common finding in inflammatory conditions. In its mild form there may be slight blunting of normally sharp carinal edges and blurring or loss of the prominent contours of bronchial cartilages (Plates 54 to 56). With marked inflammatory swelling there may be appreciable narrowing of bronchi of small calibre.

Secretions

Normal mucosa produces only sufficient clear mucus for cleansing purposes and the presence of enough to enable a sucker specimen to be obtained denotes abnormality. Such secretions vary widely, from excess of normal clear mucus in simple chronic bronchitis to frank pus in severe infections or purulent bronchitis (Plates 53, 54, 56, 57, 59 to 61 & 63). Rarely, usually in cases of asthma, thick tenacious, mucoid but viscid material may be found. This may plug the smaller (and sometimes larger) bronchi to produce obstruction and consequent pulmonary collapse. Such material may be quite beyond the patient's capacity to expectorate, but larger local plugs often can be removed by sucker or forceps (Plate 62). The patient benefits greatly from such attention and pulmonary reexpansion can be obtained. Bronchial lavage can remove more generalised secretions plugging smaller bronchi. Postoperative pulmonary deflation, due to bronchial plugging by viscid secretion, can also be quickly and adequately reexpanded by bronchoscopic sucking and inflation (Plate 60). Thin frothy secretions may occur in patients who have not received the usual atropine premedication. Such secretions, if copious and slightly pink, suggest pulmonary oedema.

The commonest secretions seen, however, are the excessive mucoid, found in simple chronic bronchitis (Plate 183). The source is the hypertrophied mucus-secreting glands present in this condition. The dilated ducts are commonly seen, particularly on the medial walls of the main bronchi just beyond the carina and on the inferior bronchial walls just within the upper lobe orifices (Plates 58, 130, 179 & 181). In severe bronchitis the secretions often become more or less purulent, but neither the degree of purulence of the secretion nor its quantity—which on occasion may be remarkable and appear almost to fill both main bronchi—are strictly related to the degree of reddening of the mucosa. Although usually occurring together, generalised reddening can be present with little increase in secretion, while considerable secretion may need aspirating from a bronchial tree with only minimal mucosal reddening. On the other hand it is quite unusual to find swelling of the mucosa without increased secretion, although in such cases reddening may be minimal.

Localised changes

Chronic bronchitis is the usual cause of generalised inflammatory changes. A localised reaction, however, raises a number of diagnostic possibilities such as carcinoma, simple pneumonia, lung abscess, tuberculosis, bronchiectasis and, less common (but often missed before bronchoscopy), inhaled foreign body. Localised inflammatory changes must not be accepted without an adequate explanation:

bronchial cancers often produce inflammatory changes in their immediate vicinity even though invisible themselves. This is such a common occurrence that it is reasonable to suspect this diagnosis in the case of localised change until proved otherwise; always provided that a careful bronchoscopic examination has excluded, as far as possible, an unsuspected foreign body (Plates 66 to 68).

If of long standing, local irritation can also lead to marked irregularity of the mucosa and finally granulation tissue, particularly well seen round foreign bodies (Plates 217 & 218). Local ulceration may also be found. This strongly suggests carcinoma but occurs with foreign bodies and in tuberculosis.

Fibrous scarring, with contractive narrowing of a bronchial orifice (Plates 94 to 96) can occur with the healing of local inflammation or ulceration, particularly tuberculosis. Scarring is also seen after radiotherapy (Plates 208, 211 & 212). The scarred areas themselves are covered with pale mucosa but the surrounding vessels may be prominent and tortuous.

As in bronchitis, the findings in bronchiectasis can vary greatly. The mucosal changes may be those of inflammation with a tendency to bleed (Plates 64 & 65), thickening or some atrophy. There may be a foul purulent discharge present (Plate 63), mucopurulent or mucoid secretion, or a dry mucosa (Plates 123 to 125). Possible anatomical changes are discussed in Chapter 7. In some cases only bronchography will reveal the disease, bronchoscopy suggesting normality.

Associated changes

Certain additional changes in the bronchial wall are commonly seen in bronchitic and emphysematous patients, particularly when symptoms of respiratory obstruction are present. Submucosal atrophy has already been mentioned in Chapter 5 as a normal ageing process but reduction of the deeper tissues, the elastic or muscle fibres, in the posterior membranous wall of the major airways has great clinical significance. Normally this membrane contracts on expiration to maintain a smooth, nearly circular contour to the bronchial lumen (Plates 13 & 14). In emphysematous patients, however, there often is loss of muscular and elastic tone, in addition to the abnormal intrathoracic pressure gradients existing in this condition. Thus marked forward displacement occurs on expiration and the lumen becomes a crescentic slit (Plates 69 to 75 & 81). Such changes can lead to severe expiratory obstruction in some patients. Similar changes can occur higher in the trachea, but they are less obvious and only rarely cause obstruction (Plate 76).

Although sometimes poorly seen in the extended, flaccid membranous wall (Plates 75 & 76), apparent hypertrophy of the elastic bundles is common, causing very prominent longitudinal mucosal corrugations. These are usually most obvious in the posterior membranous wall of the lower trachea and main bronchi (Plates 69, 70, 73 & 81). Often the ridges branch prominently into the right upper bronchus, forming a useful indicator for its location (Plate 50). Some cases of chronic bronchitis exhibit very prominent corrugations, frequently to the limit of visibility. These are particularly well seen in the lower bronchi, often with added irregularity and thickening of the overlying mucosa and submucosa. Loose, and sometimes voluminous, mucosal folds may then encroach upon the bronchial lumen. One cannot be certain, bronchoscopically, whether true hypertrophy of submucosal tissues has taken place or whether inflammatory swelling accounts for the change. There may be marked bronchial narrowing which, nevertheless, allows passage of the bronchoscope because the lining is lax and distensible, contrasting with the rigid narrowing often produced by cancer. There is further collapse on expiration with marked increase in corrugation of the mucosa (Plates 77 to 80). It is easy to visualise the mechanics of expiratory airflow obstruction, or 'air trapping', in such cases, particularly if circular muscle tissue, hypertrophied in bronchitis and even more so in asthma, contracts in 'purse-string' fashion to occlude the smaller bronchi even further.

Tuberculosis

Tuberculosis deserves special mention. It produces two main bronchoscopically visible changes: endobronchial inflammation, and distortions due to extrabronchial lymph node enlargement. One may see inflamed, swollen mucosa and purulent secretion or blood, sometimes granulomata, or even ulceration, in bronchi draining lobes or segments afflicted with active tuberculosis (Plate 84). The acute inflammatory changes can respond rapidly and visibly to chemotherapeutic treatment, leaving normal bronchi, but healing may lead to bronchial scarring and sometimes marked contractive stenosis (Plates 95 & 96). Such scarring is sometimes a surprise finding in patients with a probable history of tuberculosis, which must be the presumed cause of the stenosis (Plate 94).

Miliary tuberculosis may be seen in the mucosa and presents a similar picture to the miliary deposits sometimes seen in carcinomatosis or sarcoidosis (Plates 82, 143 & 206).

In primary tuberculosis, and occasionally in more chronic forms, gross tracheobronchial lymph node enlargement may take place (Plate 85). Overlying and adjacent mucosa may be involved to give swelling, irregularity, nodulation or local miliary deposits (Plates 82 & 83). Tuberculous granulation tissue may erupt through the mucosa to form a tumour-like mass (Plate 86). Marked distortion of the bronchial tree can occur in such cases and if the nodes caseate they may point and discharge intrabronchially. Following discharge, healing is usually steady and symptomless if the patient is receiving adequate chemotherapy. The swollen nodes subside, allowing the distorted bronchi to return to a normal pattern, while the resultant fistulae usually heal slowly, leaving small, sometimes pigmented, pitted scars in the bronchial wall (Plates 87 to 92). In many cases, the caseous nodes do not rupture but inspissate, contract and calcify, giving no further trouble. They may, however, produce ominous, irregular swellings into the main bronchi or trachea suggesting malignant invasion of lymph nodes: but the calcification seen on radiography, the usually healthy overlying mucosa and the stony hardness found on attempting biopsy, will reveal the true situation (Plate 93). Occasionally such calcifications may later begin to ulcerate through the bronchial wall to produce repeated haemoptyses. A partially extruded calcific particle (broncholith) can sometimes be removed bronchoscopically if not expectorated by the patient. This must not be tackled lightly, however, because of possible haemorrhage.

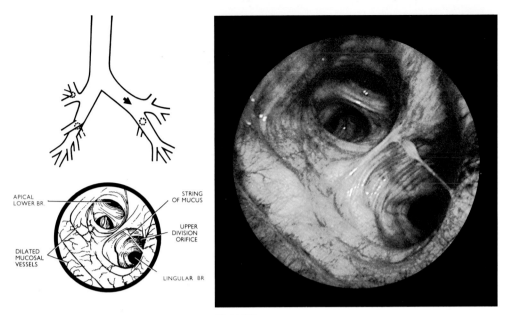

Plate 53

Chronic bronchitis. Increased vascularity, left main bronchus. Most secretions have been removed but a string persists across the upper bronchial orifice. The mucosa is generally reddened but, in addition, there is dilatation of the mucosal vessels to form a coarse, prominent network. Although widespread in the bronchial tree, the pattern was not uniformly distributed, becoming more prominent on the walls of the main and lobar bronchi. Strictly *localised* vessel prominence, in contradistinction to that described here, must always raise the suspicion of some underlying pathological process, particularly carcinoma. (Compare Plate 142.)

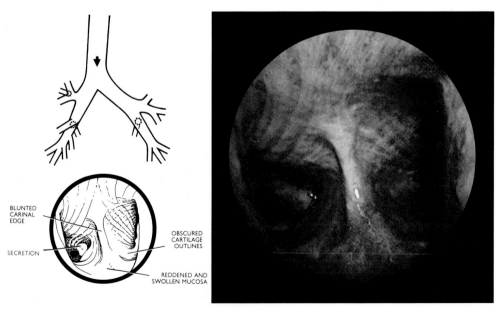

Plate 54

Chronic bronchitis. Main bifurcation. The mucosa is generally reddened and some swelling is evident: cartilage outlines are less well-defined than usual. Some increase in mucoid secretion is present, seen distally in the right main bronchus. Longitudinal mucosal corrugations are clearly visible on the posterior bronchial and tracheal walls. Bronchoscopy was performed for right middle lobe collapse following a recent bronchitic exacerbation. Removal of the obstructing secretions led to rapid recovery.

73

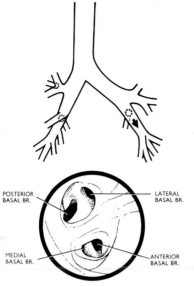
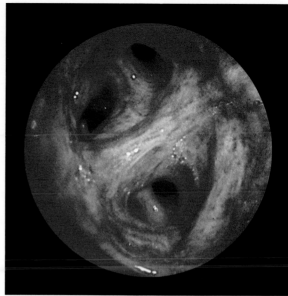

Plate 55

Bronchitis. Left basal bronchi. The changes of bronchitis are often seen to extend to the more peripheral bronchi and commonly are very marked in the basal branches where secretions readily collect. Here, mucopus has been removed to reveal the diffuse mucosal reddening and vessel engorgement. Swelling has also blurred the usually sharp outlines of the secondary carinae at this level. (Compare Plate 32.) This patient was bronchoscoped following a small haemoptysis. No other pathology was found and the very inflamed bronchial mucosa was assumed to be the source of the bleeding: a not uncommon situation in chronic bronchitis.

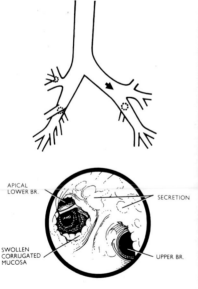
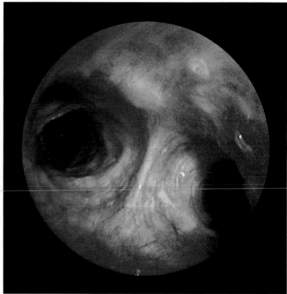

Plate 56

Bronchitis: Division of left main bronchus. The anatomy is normal with a prominent apical lower orifice visible. There is generalised reddening and vessel engorgement with increased mucus secretion, particularly noticeable on the posterior wall of the main bronchus. The mucosa is swollen and patulous, exaggerating the longitudinal corrugations, so often distributed circumferentially at this level, on the anterior wall of the lower bronchus.

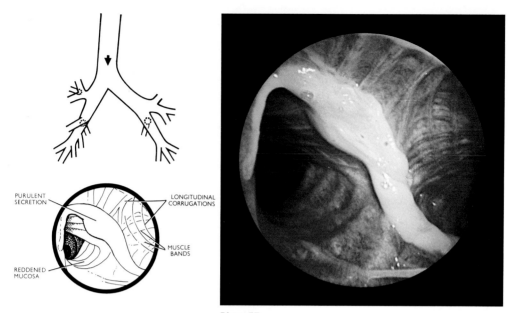

Plate 57

Bronchitis. Main bifurcation. The main feature in this case was the copious, tenacious, purulent secretion throughout the bronchial tree, here shown partially cleared to carinal level by coughing. Often such secretions are removed only with great difficulty, even with a wide bore sucker tube. The aspirating channel of the standard fibrescope was useless in this case. The mucosa is reddened, while vessels and longitudinal corrugations are prominent, so common in cases of chronic bronchitis.

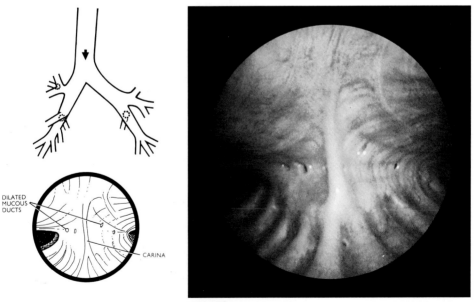

Plate 58

Bronchitis. Carina. In this case there are moderate mucosal reddening and increased vascularity, but no obvious swelling or undue prominence of the longitudinal corrugations. The main feature is the evident source of the increased mucopurulent secretion, already removed; four very obvious dilated ducts associated with the usual hypertrophy of the mucus-secreting glands. (Compare Plates 130 & 181.)

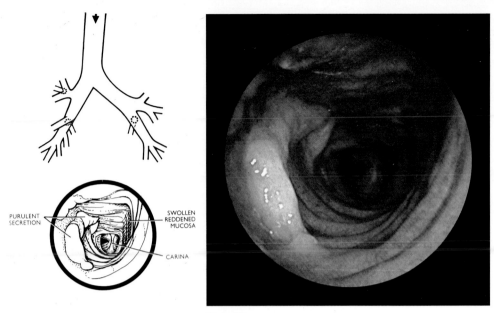

Plate 59

Bronchitis. Trachea. The carina can be seen in the distance. The mucosa is markedly reddened and sufficiently swollen to blur the cartilage outlines. Mucopurulent secretion lies in the gutter at the junction of cartilages and posterior membranous wall. It is sufficiently tenacious to adhere to the proximal lateral tracheal wall and was removed only with difficulty via a wide bore aspirating tube. This patient was considerably disabled by dyspnoea, cough and tenacious sputum; he had smoked approximately one third of a million cigarettes. The longitudinal elastic bundles are not prominent enough to corrugate the mucosa but some transverse ridging is visible in the posterior wall.

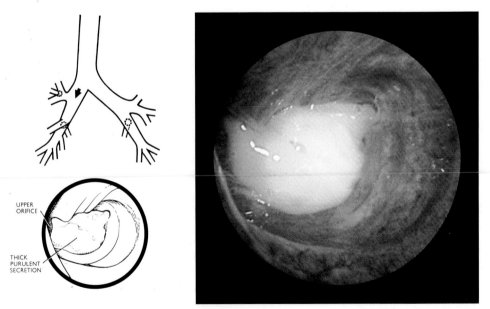

Plate 60

Postoperative pulmonary infection and collapse due to bronchial plugging. Right main bronchus. The mucosa is reddened and swollen. There is a large plug of purulent secretion blocking the lower part of the right main bronchus. The patient was too ill after laparotomy to cough adequately. Physiotherapy was not effective. Removal of the plug and secretions at bronchoscopy allowed re-expansion of the middle and lower lobes. (Compare Plates 195, 215 & 216.)

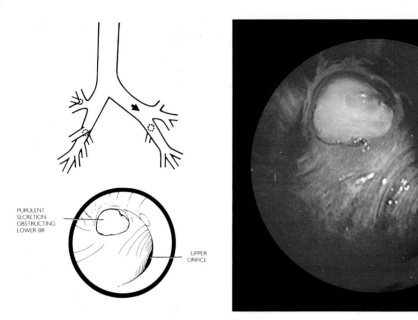

Plate 61

Pulmonary abscess. Division of left main bronchus. This is the same patient as in Plate 224. Radiography revealed an abscess in the apical lower pulmonary segment. There were generalised marked inflammatory changes throughout the bronchial tree consequent upon infection following his tracheostomy. The reddening, particularly marked on the left, is well shown here. Obstructing the lower bronchus is copious, very tenacious, thick pus which was removed with forceps and sucker. This led to rapid improvement in the patient's condition and resolution of the abscess.

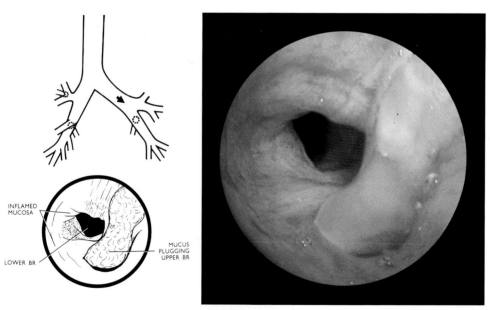

Plate 62

Asthma. Mucus plugging left upper bronchus. Bronchoscopy was indicated for increased dyspnoea with cough and total collapse of the left upper lobe, revealed radiographically. The cause is a thick, tenacious plug of mucus firmly stuck in the left upper bronchial orifice. This was removed with forceps after the large-bore sucker proved inadequate. As is usual in anaesthetised asthmatics, the bronchial wall is flaccid, and the mucosa shows generalised reddening and swelling. Additional inflammatory reaction has further narrowed the upper bronchus. The upper lobe re-expanded uneventfully.

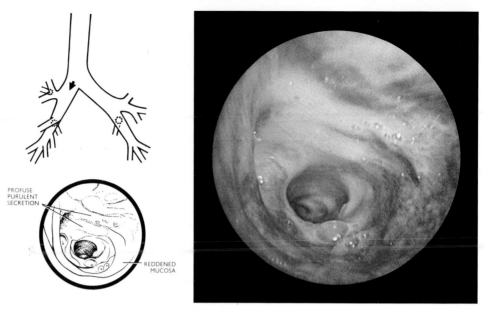

Plate 63

Purulent bronchiectasis of right basal bronchi. Right main bronchus. Copious pus is exuding from the infected basal bronchi and producing a secondary inflammatory reaction in the main bronchus: the left bronchial tree showed mild bronchitic changes only. (Compare Plates 64 & 123 to 125.)

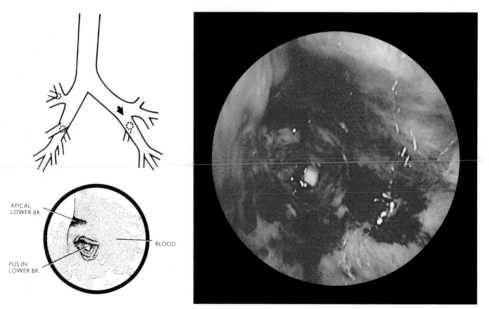

Plate 64

Left basal bronchiectasis. Left lower bronchus. In this case there is not only purulent secretion present in the basal bronchi, but the mucosa is so inflamed that it bled very readily. The patient complained of spontaneous haemoptysis as well as cough and purulent sputum. Even gentle use of the sucker has produced additional bleeding. (Compare Plates 63 & 123 to 125.)

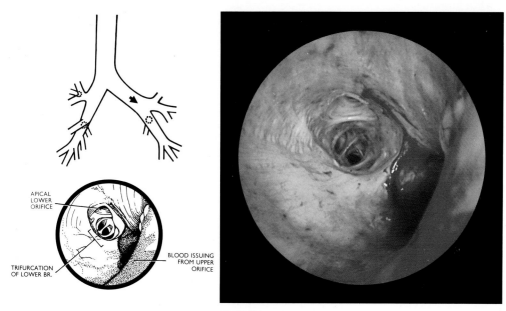

Plate 65

Bronchiectasis. Division of left main bronchus. The patient presented with repeated haemoptyses. The anatomy of the lower bronchus can be seen clearly. Fresh, partially clotted blood is oozing from the upper bronchus. After removal it became clear that this was coming from the inferior branch of the lingular bronchus. No other abnormality was found. Bronchography confirmed bronchiectasis of the inferior lingular branches and lingulectomy was performed. Bronchoscopy for further haemoptysis one year later revealed a partially extruded suture: its removal cured the symptom. (Compare Plates 233 & 234.)

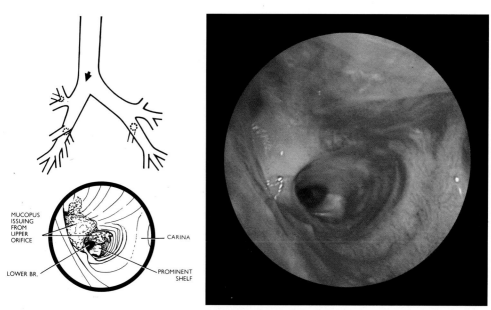

Plate 66

Localised infection. Right upper bronchus. In the left bronchial tree the mucosa was normal and no secretion was present. Round the right upper orifice, however, the mucosa was reddened and swollen, and issuing from the orifice was purulent secretion, here seen flowing down the intermediate bronchus. This was easily removed, revealing an otherwise normal orifice. These findings and the absence of malignant cells in the sputum, supported the clinical diagnosis of simple pulmonary infection in the right upper lobe. Prompt resolution followed antibiotic therapy. (Compare Plates 67 & 68.)

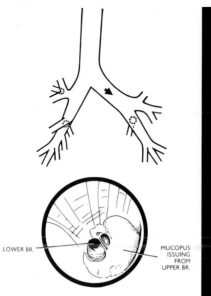

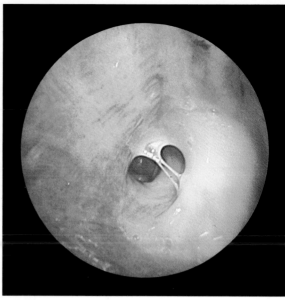

LOWER BR.

MUCOPUS
ISSUING
FROM
UPPER BR.

Plate 67

Localised infection. Left upper bronchus. The patient presented with a picture suggesting left upper lobe pneumonia. There was a slow, poor response to antimicrobial therapy and bronchial carcinoma was suspected. Copious purulent material is seen exuding from the left upper orifice. The mucosa within this bronchus was found reddened and swollen after removing the secretion. No other evidence of tumour was obtained bronchoscopically: sucker and swab specimens contained no malignant cells and biopsy of the inflamed mucosa was negative. Radiological changes remained suspicious of bronchial carcinoma in the anterior segment of the upper lobe and subsequent thoracotomy and lobectomy confirmed this. Histology: oat-cell carcinoma. A case of localised infection secondary to a malignant process, itself beyond bronchoscopic vision. (Compare Plates 66 & 68.)

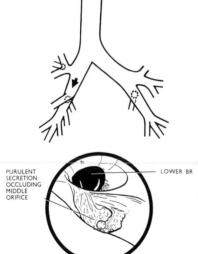

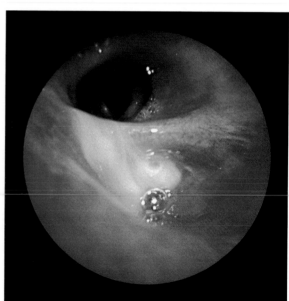

PURULENT
SECRETION
OCCLUDING
MIDDLE
ORIFICE

LOWER BR

Plate 68

Localised infection. Right middle bronchus. Cough, sputum, and middle lobe collapse, in a heavy cigarette smoker aged 60 years, aroused suspicion of bronchial carcinoma. The locally reddened, swollen mucosa, producing luminal narrowing of the middle bronchus just beyond its orifice, and the plugging with purulent secretion, both indicated a local inflammatory reaction possibly secondary to carcinoma. Absence of malignant cells in the sucker and swab specimens, a biopsy showing inflammatory reaction only, and lobar re-expansion following a week of antibiotic treatment and physiotherapy, all indicated simple local infection. The patient was still well six months later. (Compare Plates 66 & 67.)

80

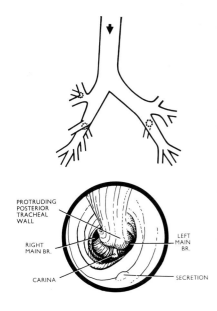

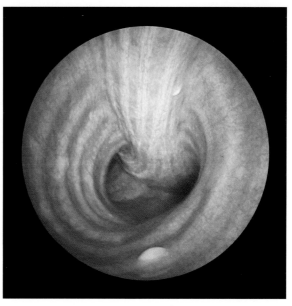

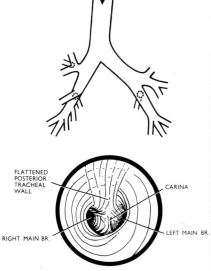

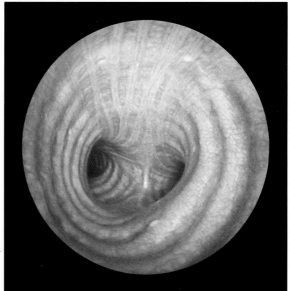

Plates 69 & 70

Chronic bronchitis. Loss of tone in posterior tracheal wall. This patient had stopped smoking for some years, hence the relatively normal mucosa and only minimal secretion, but the flaccidity of the posterior tracheal and main bronchial walls persists, with prominent longitudinal corrugations. In the relaxed unconscious patient (Plate 69) this membrane is bulging forward sufficiently to obscure the carina and reduce the lumina, making them crescent-shaped in section. This general loss of tone is commonly seen in bronchitic patients and the characteristic distortion is very reminiscent of a mole-run. It occurs on only slight expiratory effort or even in the relaxed condition: coughing would be needed to produce a similar effect in normal subjects. This degree of forward protrusion may suggest a pathological cause posterior to the lower trachea but, raising the intrabronchial pressure, either by inspiration or ventilation, will rapidly abolish any doubt: the flaccid membrane is immediately extended and a circular bronchial outline restored (Plate 70). Rigid tissues, or posterior lymph node enlargement, will prevent this effect. (Compare Plates 13, 14, 71 to 74, 97, 98 & 102.)

81

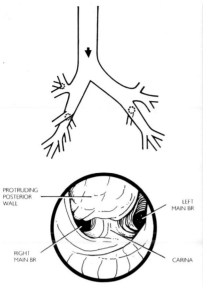

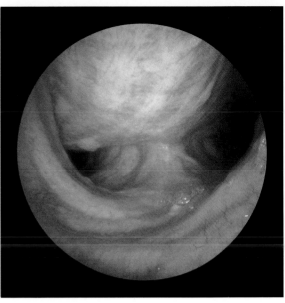

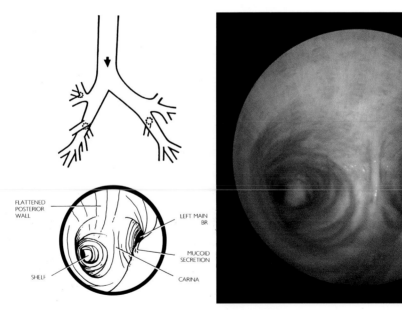

Plates 71 & 72

Chronic bronchitis. Loss of tone in posterior tracheal and main bronchial walls. The findings are very similar to those in Plates 69 and 70, but the continuation of the flaccidity into both main bronchi, particularly the right, is more obvious. Here the bronchial lumen is considerably reduced in the relaxed state (Plate 71) and remarkably increased on inflation (Plate 72). The longitudinal corrugations are well seen, the mucosa is rather reddened and there is some increase in secretion. A 'shelf' is clearly visible in the distance in Plate 72. (Compare Plates 16, 42, 43, 69, 70, 73, 74, 97, 98 & 102.)

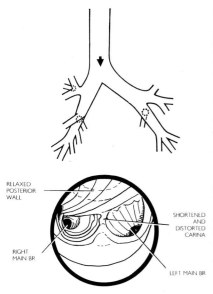

RELAXED POSTERIOR WALL

RIGHT MAIN BR

SHORTENED AND DISTORTED CARINA

LEFT MAIN BR

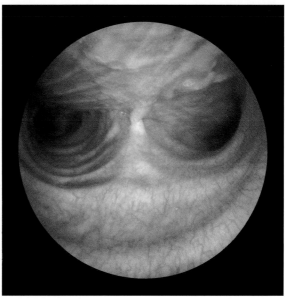

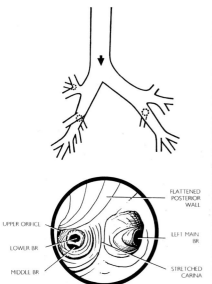

FLATTENED POSTERIOR WALL

UPPER ORIFICE

LOWER BR

MIDDLE BR

LEFT MAIN BR

STRETCHED CARINA

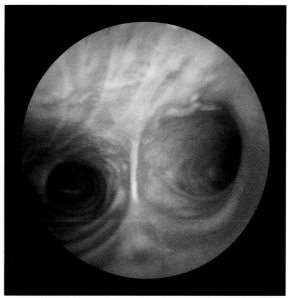

Plates 73 & 74

Chronic bronchitis. Loss of tone. In this case the flaccidity of the posterior tracheal wall is not so marked as in Plates 69 to 72. Thus in the relaxed state the carina is not obscured and its change in shape clearly can be seen: folded and thickened in Plate 73, stretched and knife-like in Plate 74. There is the usual prominence of the longitudinal corrugations, some mucosal reddening and an increase in secretion. In addition to the chronic bronchitis, a left-sided carcinoma was also found. (Compare Plates 69 to 72, 97, 98 & 102.)

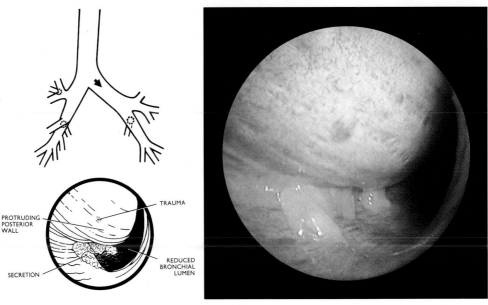

Plate 75

Chronic bronchitis. Excessive secretion and loss of tone: posterior wall of left main bronchus (same patient as Plate 76). Here there is definite protrusion of the membranous wall but the posterior longitudinal corrugations are not prominent. There was copious mucopurulent secretion present, some of which has been removed by sucking: hence the small traumatic ecchymosis in the posterior bronchial wall.

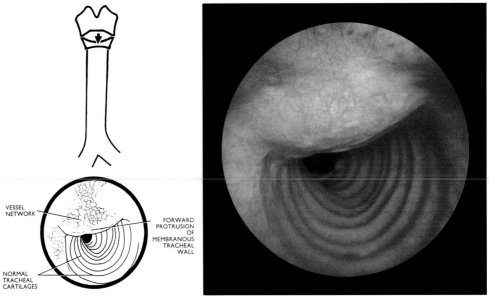

Plate 76

Chronic bronchitis. Loss of tone in trachea. The posterior membranous wall is bulging forward into the lumen. Frequently the atony and flaccidity responsible for this are only demonstrable in the lower intrathoracic part of the trachea but, in this case, the change is clearly seen in the upper third: it was present throughout the trachea and main bronchi in this patient (see Plate 75). The posterior longitudinal mucosal corrugations have disappeared, presumably with degeneration of the elastic bundles, and a fine vascular network can be made out in the slightly reddened mucosa. (Compare Plate 173.)

84

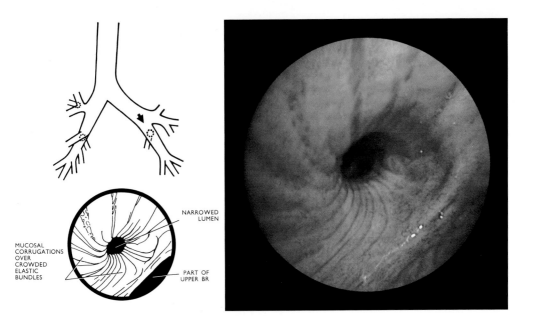

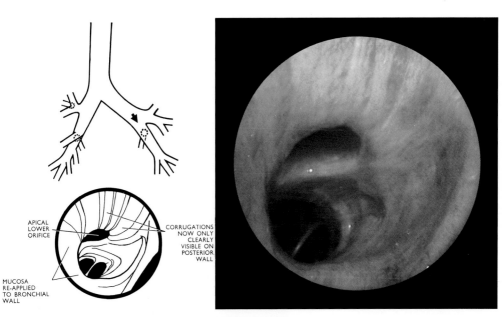

Plates 77 & 78

Chronic bronchitis. Left lower bronchus. Secretions have been removed but the mucosa is swollen and reddened. The upper picture is taken in the relaxed unconscious patient: in the lower the intraluminal pressure has been increased by using the ventilator. Although the lumen is narrowed by mucosal swelling, flaccidity and hypertrophy of elements in its wall, it is also distensible and passes the bronchoscope easily during relaxation under anaesthesia. It is easy to see, however, that complete closure could take place on moderate expiratory effort which would force the inner bronchial wall still further away from its cartilagenous support. The hypertrophied longitudinal elastic bundles are prominent and, at this level, are seen to surround the bronchial lumen: they become much less obvious when the lumen is distended. If muscle hypertrophy also is present, as in asthma, the condition may be exaggerated still further. (Compare Plates 79 & 80.)

85

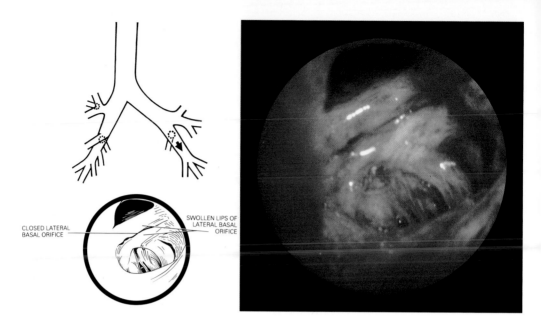

CLOSED LATERAL
BASAL ORIFICE

SWOLLEN LIPS OF
LATERAL BASAL
ORIFICE

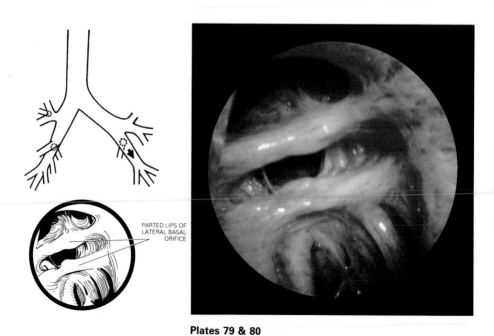

PARTED LIPS OF
LATERAL BASAL
ORIFICE

Plates 79 & 80

Chronic bronchitis. Left basal bronchi. This patient was a heavy smoker with a long history of chronic cough. This had increased recently. Bronchoscopy revealed a carcinoma of the right upper bronchus in addition to the generalised changes of chronic bronchitis. The mucosal flaccidity and swelling were particularly noticable in the left basal bronchi, here depicted in relaxation (Plate 79) and during inflation with the ventilator (Plate 80). (Compare Plates 77 & 78.)

86

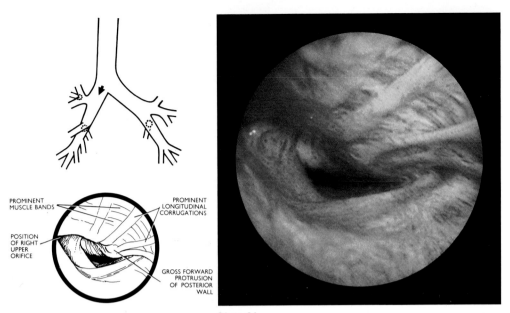

Plate 81

Chronic bronchitis. Loss of tone in right main bronchus. There is general reddening, swelling and increased vascularity, but the most impressive feature is the gross forward protrusion of the flaccid posterior membrane, which immediately flattened on pulmonary inflation. Both the prominent longitudinal corrugations and the muscle bundles are very well demonstrated. On the far left of the picture the effect is seen to extend into the upper bronchus. (Compare Plate 151.)

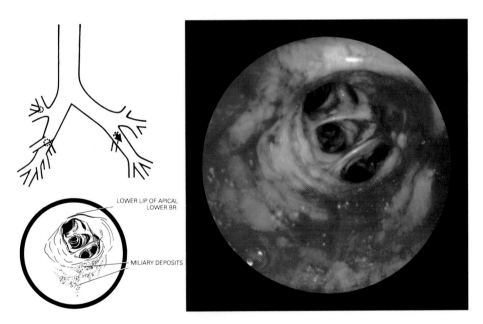

Plate 82

Tuberculosis. Left lower bronchus. Cough for some months, followed by haemoptysis, led to bronchoscopy. The lower lip of the apical lower bronchus is seen at the picture periphery; the basal bronchi distally. Some blood is present, partially obscuring miliary deposits in the anterior bronchial wall mucosa. Tubercle bacilli were grown from the bronchial aspirate. (Compare Plates 143 & 206.)

87

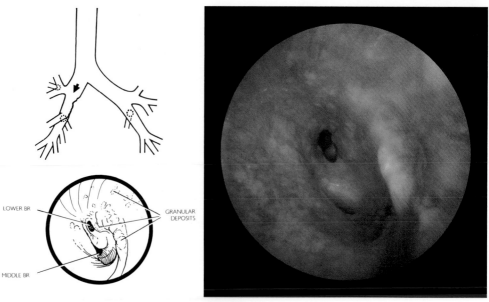

Plate 83

Tuberculosis. Right intermediate bronchus. This patient presented with a history of malaise and weight loss for three months and a productive cough for one month. There had been contact with a tuberculous patient six months previously. The chest radiograph showed bilateral hilar and upper mediastinal lymphadenopathy with some diffuse nodular shadowing in the lung fields. There is generalized reddening and swelling of the mucosa. The medial bronchial wall is displaced laterally by node enlargement. The overlying mucosa is thickened, irregular and nodular. Smaller, discrete, pale nodules are also present on the posterior wall. Sputum culture yielded tubercle bacilli: mucosal biopsy showed multiple granulomata, typical of tuberculosis.

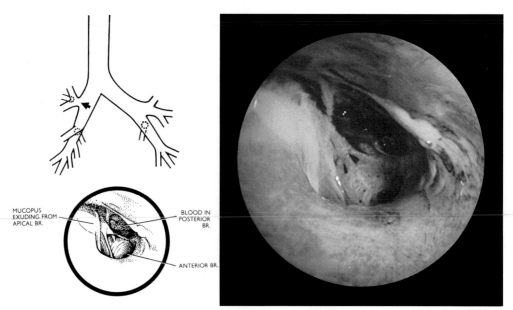

Plate 84

Tuberculosis. Right upper bronchus. Lateral-viewing telescope. Cough, haemoptysis, pleuritic chest pain and right upper zone shadowing in the radiograph led to bronchoscopy after sputum examination proved negative. Fresh blood is seen to be issuing from the posterior segmental orifice; mucopus from the apical. The aspirate yielded tubercle bacilli. Chemotherapy led to steady and complete recovery.

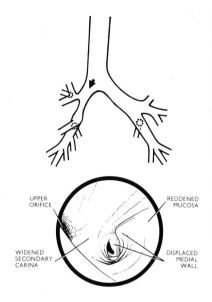

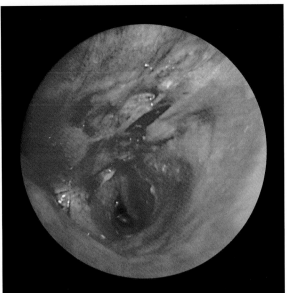

Plate 85

Active tuberculous lymphadenitis. Right main bronchus. The mucosa is markedly reddened and swollen. The medial wall of the main bronchus is displaced laterally and the secondary carina between main and upper bronchi is widened; both changes are due to lymph node enlargement. In consequence the lumen of the lower part of the right main bronchus is greatly reduced and the upper orifice is narrowed. Bleeding occurred readily from slight trauma. Biopsy: typical histology of active tuberculosis; tubercle bacilli grew on culture.

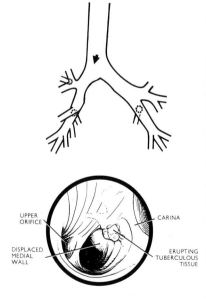

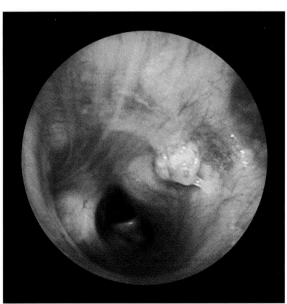

Plate 86

Active tuberculous lymphadenitis. Carina and right main bronchus. The patient presented with persistent cough, lassitude and enlarged upper mediastinal shadow in the radiograph. There is a minor increase in mucosal vascular markings. The medial and postero-medial walls of the main bronchus are protruding into the lumen due to underlying lymph node enlargement. Just beyond the widened carina, granulation tissue is erupting through the mucosa. Biopsy: typical tuberculous histology with acid-fast bacilli present.

89

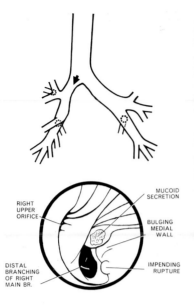

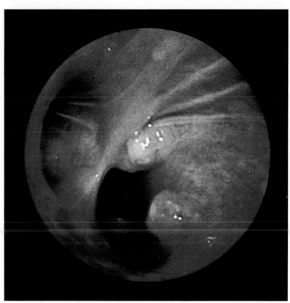

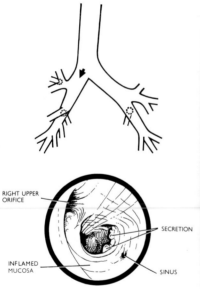

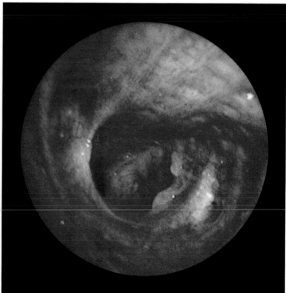

Plates 87 & 88

Tuberculosis lymphadenitis: intrabronchial rupture. Right main bronchus. The patient presented with lassitude, weight loss, persistent cough and wheeze, all of recent onset. Plate 87 illustrates gross suppurative enlargement of the subcarinal lymph nodes. The resulting swelling is thrusting into the right main bronchus through its medial wall. The consequent displacement of the posterior mucosal corrugations and the point of impending rupture are both seen clearly. There is secretion lying on the posterior wall and the entrance to the upper bronchus is unusually prominent. The same point in the bronchial tree, re-photographed after nine months of continuous antituberculosis chemotherapy, is illustrated in Plate 88. Spontaneous rupture has occurred at the expected place and·a fistula now exists, which discharged a small quantity of clear tenacious fluid. The mucosa remains reddened, but anatomical relations have been restored to normality. (See also Plates 89 & 90.)

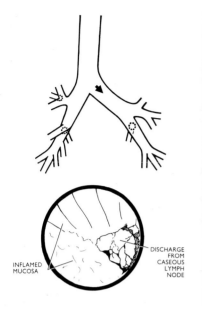

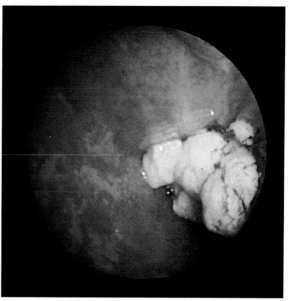

INFLAMED MUCOSA

DISCHARGE FROM CASEOUS LYMPH NODE

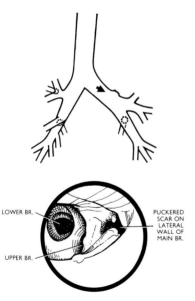

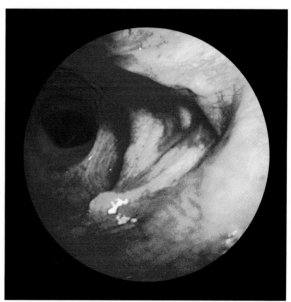

LOWER BR.

UPPER BR.

PUCKERED SCAR ON LATERAL WALL OF MAIN BR.

Plates 89 & 90

Tuberculous lymphadenitis: intrabronchial rupture. Left main bronchus. This is the same case as illustrated in Plates 87 and 88: the photographs were taken at the same times. In addition to the subcarinal node enlargement another large node was present lateral to the left main bronchus. This ruptured while the bronchoscope was in place, discharging its caseous contents intrabronchially (Plate 89). This was easily removed with the sucker. Plate 90 shows the puckered and pigmented residual scar after nine months chemotherapy. Although the mucosa remains reddened and there is some mucoid secretion, the patient was symptomless and fit.

91

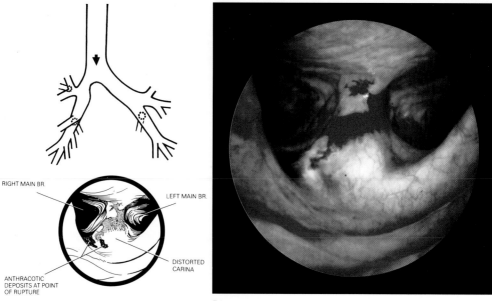

Plate 91

Tuberculosis lymphadenitis: intrabronchial rupture. This 85-year-old man gave a history of cough with grey sputum for three months and one episode of haemoptysis. Sputum culture yielded tubercle bacilli. Two sisters had died of tuberculosis in youth. The carina is widened anteriorly by an enlarged subcarinal node. Secretions have been removed to reveal the point of node rupture and an anthracotic deposit. Fresh blood lies on the carina. A case of recrudescence of lymph node infection, presumably contracted in youth. (Compare Plates 87 to 90.)

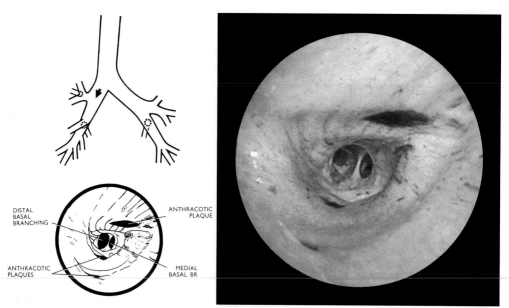

Plate 92

Anthracotic deposits. Right main bronchus. Hard, depressed, black plaques are occasionally seen in the major bronchi. Although it is rare to be able to establish their origin in an individual case, they have been observed to follow intrabronchial perforation of tuberculosis lymph nodes. (Compare Plate 90.) The black pigment derives from anthracotic material, present in the nodes, which is subsequently incorporated in the scarred areas. In this case there are three well-defined, anthracotic plaques in the right main bronchus. As isolated, incidental findings they have no further clinical significance. Small flecks of haemorrhage are also present in this case due to slight sucker trauma. (Compare Plates 177 & 189.) Similar plaques may be found in coal miners. (See Plate 229.)

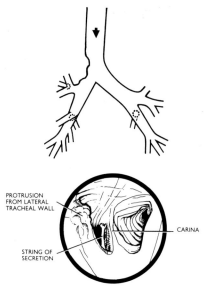

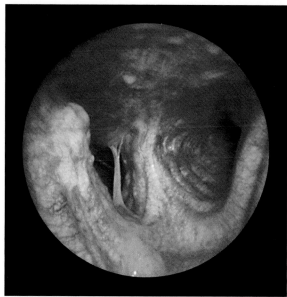

PROTRUSION
FROM LATERAL
TRACHEAL WALL

CARINA

STRING OF
SECRETION

Plate 93

Tuberculosis. Calcified paratracheal node. Bronchoscopy was undertaken for minor haemoptysis. The inflammatory changes present are those of chronic bronchitis with mucosal reddening and vessel engorgement. Tenacious mucopurulent secretion is seen in the right main bronchus. There is a minor anatomical variation in the shape of the carina. (Compare Plates 48 & 198.) On the right, lateral, lower tracheal wall there is a craggy projection, paler than the surrounding mucosa. Superficially it resembled tumour tissue but was impossible to biopsy because of its very hard consistency. Not seen on the PA radiograph, this calcified paratracheal node was subsequently confirmed on the lateral film. It was not clear whether the bleeding was from the bronchitic mucosa or due to the broncholith. Attempts at bronchoscopic removal of such broncholiths can lead to profuse haemorrhage and are best avoided. (Compare Plate 134.)

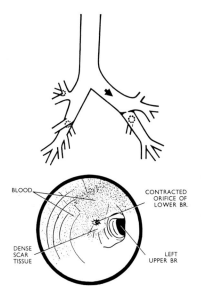

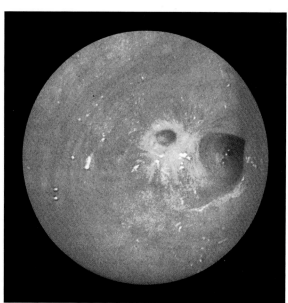

BLOOD

CONTRACTED
ORIFICE OF
LOWER BR.

DENSE
SCAR
TISSUE

LEFT
UPPER BR.

Plate 94

Postinflammatory contractive scarring. Left lower bronchus. The orifice of the left lower bronchus has become a small rigid stricture through which it was impossible to pass even a telescope. The edges of this were avascular and pale, in contrast to the surrounding mucosa which was reddened and swollen due to chronic bronchitis. This patient had a history of left lower lobe infection 44 years previously at the age of 10 years. It was a prolonged illness and may well have been tuberculosis. He presented with repeated left lower lobe infections.

93

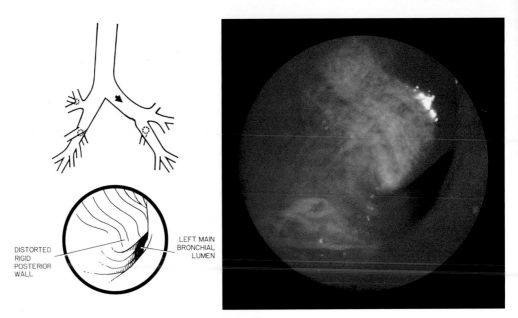

Plate 95

Post-tuberculous scarring. Left main bronchus. Many years previously, this heavily-smoking patient had suffered from extensive pulmonary tuberculosis of the left lung, chiefly affecting the upper lobe. Bronchoscopy was performed when a recent history of increased cough, sputum and haemoptysis, accompanied by new shadowing in the radiograph, raised suspicions of a carcinoma or recrudescence of tuberculosis. Mucopurulent secretion has been removed, revealing reddened, swollen mucosa and gross distortion of the posterior wall of the left main bronchus. There was also marked distortion and upward displacement of the left upper bronchus. Biopsies from the distorted area revealed no carcinoma or tuberculosis: no tubercle bacilli were found in the bronchial aspirate. The patient's symptoms responded to antimicrobial therapy and follow-up was uneventful. Diagnosis: simple superadded infection in a lung previously damaged by tuberculosis.

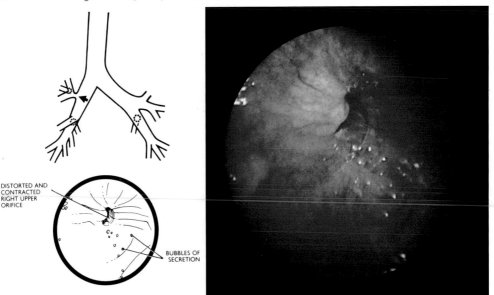

Plate 96

Post-tuberculous scarring. Right upper bronchus. Lateral-viewing telescope. This patient remained well for 20 years following treatment for right upper lobe pulmonary tuberculosis and then suffered repeated small haemoptyses. The upper orifice is seen to be greatly narrowed. It is also distorted, particularly its upper lip which shows pale, fibrous scarring. There is generalised mucosal reddening and mucoid secretion is issuing from the orifice. The narrowed lumen, and marked upward deflection of the bronchus due to lobar contraction, made it impossible to examine in depth, even with the fibrescope. Bronchography confirmed great bronchial distortion and bronchiectasis.

CHAPTER 7

BRONCHIAL DISTORTION
AND DISPLACEMENT

The trachea or bronchi may be displaced or distorted in various ways, but local compression, usually by extrabronchial pressure from enlarged tracheobronchial lymph nodes, is that most commonly seen. Any pathological process producing node enlargement can result in similar distortion, for this depends more on the degree of enlargement than on its cause: determination of the pathology will often depend on other factors, such as finding a visible, primary bronchial carcinoma, the state of the overlying bronchial mucosa (Ch. 8), or the results of investigatory procedures other than bronchoscopy. Primary tumours can also lead to local distortion and if not invasive are unlikely to affect the overlying mucosa (Plates 39 & 105).

The commonest positions for distortion to appear are those adjacent to prominent groups of lymph nodes. In particular, enlargement of the subcarinal nodes readily produces widening of this area and eventually an abolition of the usual keel-sharp edge of the carina: this is a very common confirmatory sign of the inoperability of a bronchial carcinoma (Plates 103 & 104). Frequently the size of these nodes is such that pressure on the medial wall of either or both main bronchi continues peripherally for a varying distance (Plates 103 & 119). Such pressure produces a lateral bulging of the medial wall to change the cross-section of the lumen from roughly circular to bean-shaped, crescentic or a slit (Plate 114). Extensive tumour involvement of the mediastinum, either primary or secondary, may produce a bilateral effect to considerable depth in both main and lower bronchi (Plates 107 & 108). Enlarged paratracheal nodes frequently distort and sometimes compress the trachea (Plates 99 & 100). Posteriorly placed nodes may also enlarge to produce forward bulging of posterior main bronchial (Plate 109) or tracheal (Plates 97, 98 & 102) walls and an apparent shortening and widening of the carina at this level (Plate 102). This can be distinguished from simple loss of tone of the posterior membraneous wall by the rigidity of the tissues and the persistence of the swelling on increasing the intrabronchial pressure (compare Plates 69 & 70). Compression by bronchopulmonary lymph node enlargement is also common. The orifice of the right upper bronchus may be distorted or closed by compression (Plates 85 & 111 to 113) and the secondary carina at the primary division of the left main bronchus is not uncommonly widened (Plates 117 & 118).

A particularly striking feature of local bronchial distortion is the displacement and crowding of the posterior longitudinal corrugations, if these happen to be present in the vicinity. Commonly such distortion is seen in the main bronchi, when an enlarged subcarinal node displaces a medial wall laterally (Plates 99, 106, 108 to 110, 119, 136 & 140). If the swelling is placed behind the posterior membranous wall this may be so stretched (or invaded if the tumour is malignant) that the longitudinal corrugations are obliterated, rather than simply displaced (Plates 97, 98 & 102).

Other causes of localised bronchial distortion are developmental anomalies (Plates 48 to 52), inflammatory fibrosis (Plates 94 to 96 & 218), neoplasic involvement of the bronchial wall (Ch. 8), sarcoidosis (Plates 203 & 206), radiotherapy (Plates 132 & 208) and trauma (Plates 219 & 220). Severe general distortion of the thoracic cage, such as that produced by kyphosis, can occasionally give a confusing picture (Plate 101).

Displacement of bronchi, as in the case of localised distortion, may also be due to a number of different causes. There may be generalised unilateral extrinsic pressure, such as that produced by a pleural effusion or pneumothorax, obliging the lung on that side to take up less space than usual. The consequent contraction may be obvious (Plates 115 & 116), or so uniformly spread throughout the bronchial tree that it can only be appreciated by careful comparison of bronchial calibre with the contralateral findings. More localised pressure such as that from loculated fluid or air, large cysts, tumours, phrenic paralysis or collapse therapy may produce very clear changes. For example, the right upper bronchus may swing downwards to a remarkable degree, so that its lumen can be inspected clearly from the level of the carina (Plate 126). In less florrid cases, only smaller bronchi may be distorted (Plate 127).

Collapse of pulmonary tissue without extrinsic pressure, for example in cases of bronchiectasis, can also produce obvious abnormality. The medial displacement of the left main bronchus in cases of left lower lobe collapse may be particularly striking, giving, from the lower trachea, an unusually clear view down both main bronchi simultaneously: even more pronounced if both lower lobes are deflated (Plates 120 & 121). The left upper bronchus usually swings downwards in such cases to come more in line with the main bronchus, at the expense of the medially displaced lower (Plate 122). Similarly in basal bronchiectasis all the basal bronchi on the side affected may sometimes be visualised to a considerable depth from the same viewpoint in the lower bronchus: a finding equivalent to the 'crowding' of the bronchi seen bronchographically (Plates 123 & 124). In middle lobe bronchiectasis it may be unusually easy to see, with a rigid telescope, into the bronchial lumen as far as the primary division (Plate 125).

Resection of lung tissue will lead to displacement of the bronchi as the remaining lung tissue expands to fill the residual space. In addition the bronchial stump is usually visible, presenting a puckered, irregular appearance at the point of closure (Plates 128 to 130).

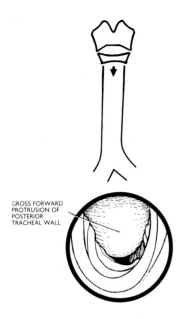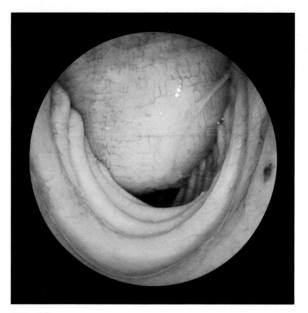

Plate 97

Tracheal compression. This patient presented with stridor and persistent, non-pleuritic, aching pain in the central chest. The radiograph revealed a large right-sided hilar mass. The gross forward displacement of the posterior tracheal wall by lymph nodes, presumably involved in carcinoma, is well seen. It has been stretched to a thin smooth membrane abolishing any suggestion of the longitudinal corrugations. The lumen is grossly reduced, but it was possible to reach the upper bronchus with the fibrescope and confirm the presence of oat-cell carcinoma in its posterior segmental branch. Radiotherapy was highly effective in returning the trachea to normality and relieving the patient of his stridor. (Compare Plates 69 to 71, 98, 102, 211 & 212.)

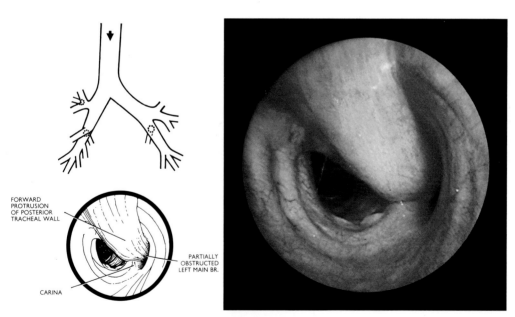

Plate 98

Tracheal distortion. Persistent wheezing, located in the left chest, and partial loss of voice were this patient's main complaints. There was left vocal cord paralysis in addition to the gross forward displacement of the posterior wall of the trachea and left main bronchus, clearly shown here. A feature is the abolition of the mucosal corrugations in the stretched mucosa, usually retained in the flaccidity of bronchitis. Both the distal left main bronchus and the distorted region were rigid: there was no change on ventilation. Biopsy of mucosa in left main bronchus: oat-cell carcinoma. (Compare Plates 69 to 71, 97 & 102.)

97

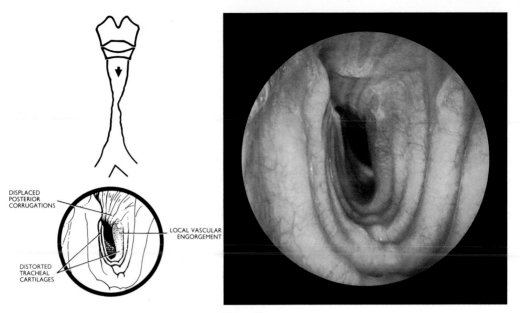

Plate 99

Compression by enlarged lymph nodes. 'Scabbard' trachea. A case of left lower bronchial carcinoma presenting with dyspnoea, due to a large left pleural effusion, and hoarseness. There were already paralysis of the left vocal cord and metastases in mediastinal, bilateral paratracheal and cervical lymph nodes. The left paratracheal mass was particularly large and accounts for the more marked medial displacement of the left tracheal wall, where the local redness indicates early involvement of the mucosa. With both walls displaced medially the tracheal shape is truly reminiscent of a scabbard. Local displacement of the posterior, longitudinal corrugations is a typical feature of distortion produced by lymph node enlargement. Biopsy from left main bronchus: oat-cell carcinoma. (Compare Plate 8.)

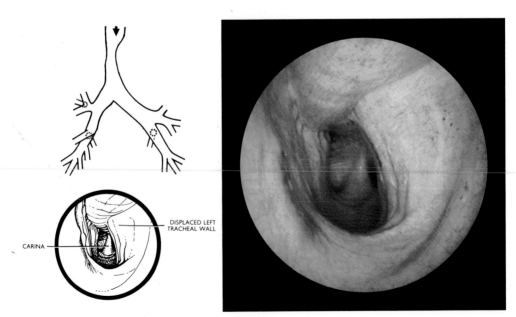

Plate 100

Distortion by enlarged lymph nodes. Trachea. The left lateral wall of the trachea is distorted by an enlarged paratracheal lymph node involved in carcinoma. The cartilage outlines have been abolished and the flaccid, protruded, posterior wall deflected laterally. In the distance, the carina appears normal but the medial wall of the right main bronchus is distorted by enlarged mediastinal nodes. Biopsy: undifferentiated carcinoma.

98

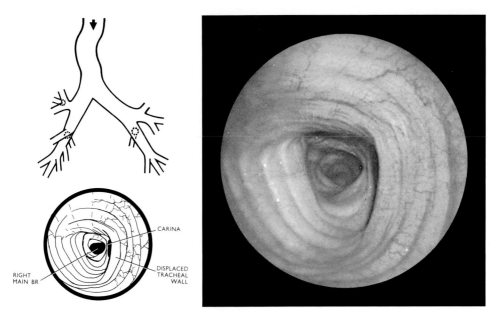

Plate 101

Tortuous trachea. The patient was elderly and had a remarkable degree of thoracic kyphosis. Since no other cause for the tracheal distortion could be found, it could only be attributed to this condition. The essential difference between this situation and that found with lymph node compression is that here the tracheal walls have remained parallel: a simple tortuosity has accompanied approximation of larynx and carina. With lymph node enlargement, displacement of the wall adjacent to the node is the more conspicuous, so producing narrowing of the lumen.

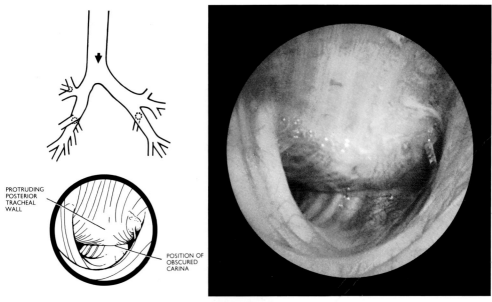

Plate 102

Lower tracheal compression. Unrelieved wheeze, cough and weight loss were the patient's main complaints. Just proximal to the carina the posterior tracheal wall is considerably displaced forward by a large metastatic deposit from an oat-cell carcinoma of the left upper bronchus. At the point of maximal forward displacement the posterior mucosal corrugations cease, and a localised smooth swelling takes their place. This largely obscures the carina and greatly reduces the lumina of the main bronchi. Increasing the intraluminal pressure did not alter the situation. (Compare Plates 69 to 71, 97 & 98.)

99

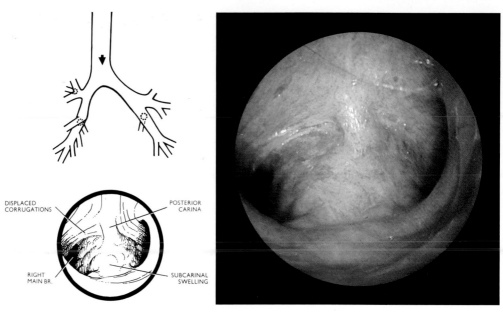

Plate 103

Carinal widening. Main bifurcation. There is extensive invasion of the subcarinal lymph nodes by metastatic tumour from a right upper bronchial carcinoma. The carinal edge has disappeared except for a short portion posteriorly. The large swelling extends distally to displace the medial walls of both main bronchi, to considerably reduce their lumina and to abolish the cartilage outlines. The overlaying mucosa is moderately reddened and a little irregular, suggesting early invasion by tumour.

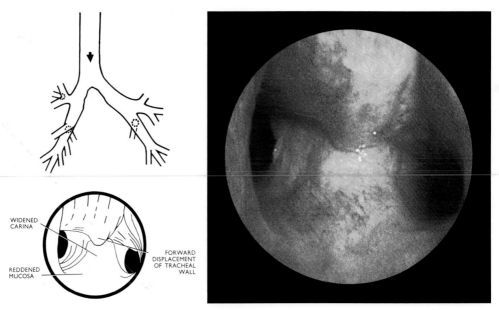

Plate 104

Carinal widening. Main bifurcation. Malignant subcarinal lymph node enlargement has blunted the carina: the sharp edge is lost and it is widened to become saddle-shaped. Just proximal to the carina an extension of the node enlargement has thrust forward a small part of the posterior tracheal wall. The mucosa is reddened and swollen. The primary tumour was an undifferentiated bronchial carcinoma beyond bronchoscopic vision and numerous other estrapulmonary metastases soon appeared.

100

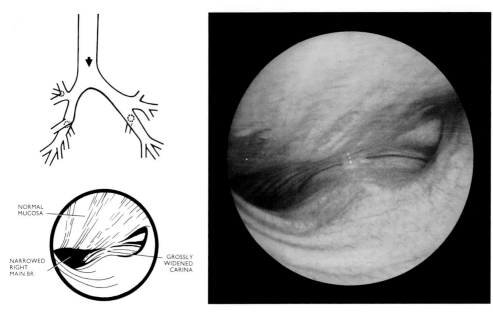

Plate 105

Carinal widening. Main birfurcation. A large benign, cystic tumour lies in the subcarinal area and has grossly distorted the carina and first part of both main bronchi. It was removed uneventfully. It is unusual for malignant subcarinal lymph node metastases to reach this size without involving the overlying mucosa in the tumour process and consequently producing irregularity or at least considerable inflammation: a benign tumour was thus suspected at bronchoscopy. The large lymph node swellings produced by sarcoidosis can show a similar picture, but usually with reddened overlying mucosa. (Compare Plates 39 & 203.)

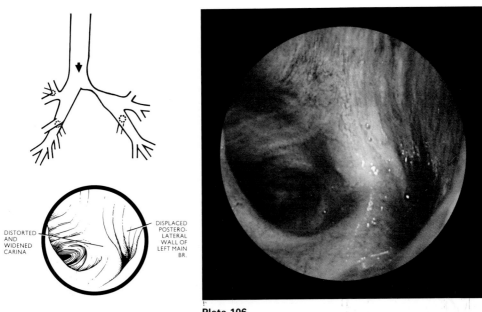

Plate 106

Compression by enlarged lymph nodes. Carina and main bronchi. The main finding was persistent, loud wheeze over the left upper chest. A left paratracheal lymph node and, to a lesser extent, a subcarinal node are secondarily involved with carcinoma arising in the left bronchial tree. The degree of distortion is such that little lumen remains in the left main bronchus and the primary growth could not be reached. The surrounding mucosa is reddened and swollen; there is mucopurulent secretion exuding from the narrowed lumen. Aspiration needle biopsy of carina: undifferentiated carcinoma.

101

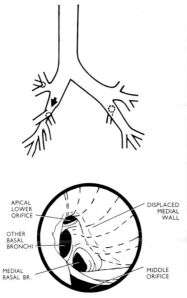

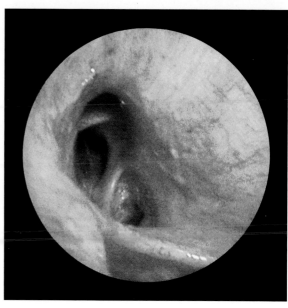

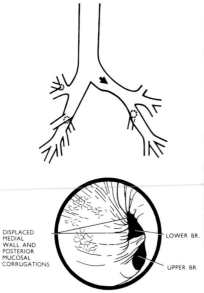

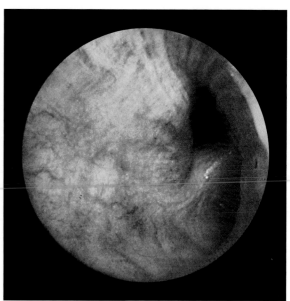

Plates 107 & 108

Compression by a large, central thoracic tumour. Right lower bronchus (Plate 107) and left main bronchus (Plate 108). The carina itself was not widened, but the size of the mass, a carcinoma originating in the left medial basal pulmonary segment and invading the mediastinum and right lower lobe, led to distortion of both right and left bronchial trees. The medial bronchial walls are thrust laterally so that the normally circular lumina are crescent-shaped. In the left main bronchus deflection of the posterior mucosal corrugations further emphasises the distortion that has occurred. The mucosa is reddened, particularly over the distorted regions.

102

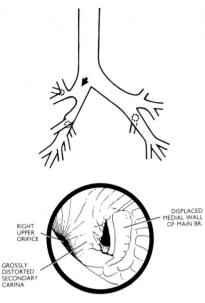

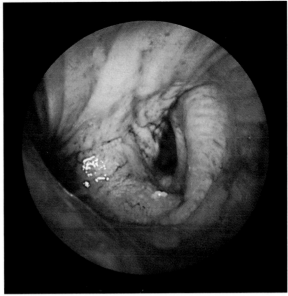

Plate 113

Distortion of secondary carina. Right main bronchus. The patient complained of persistent cough, lassitude and recent haemoptyses. The carina was widened and rigid. Seen here is the secondary carina, normally forming the lower lip of the right upper bronchus. It is grossly widened and rounded by enlarged lymph nodes and there are dilated vessels in the covering mucosa. The lumen of the intermediate bronchus is further narrowed by irregular tumour tissue displacing the longitudinal corrugations. After removing blood from the upper bronchus, tumour tissue was found therein. Biopsy: undifferentiated carcinoma. (Compare Plates 85, 111 & 112.)

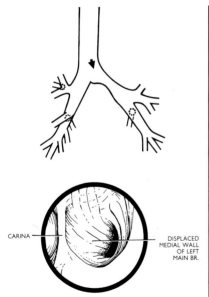

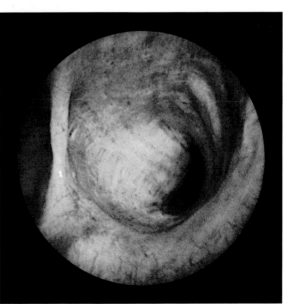

Plate 114

Distortion by enlarged lymph nodes. Left main bronchus. Unresolving pneumonia of the right lower lobe led to bronchoscopy. Although the carina is seen to be sharp, there is marked mediastinal swelling displacing the medial wall of the left main bronchus laterally. The lumen is reduced to approximately half the normal calibre. A similar situation was present on the right and there, in addition, the primary, polypoidal tumour was found arising from the basal system and obstructing the lower bronchus. Biopsy: squamous-cell carcinoma.

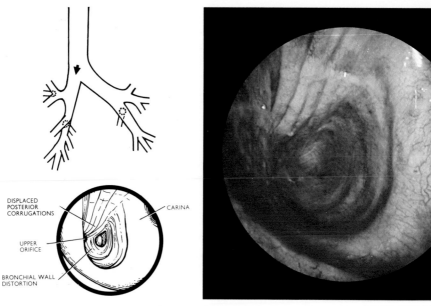

Plate 115

Right bronchial displacement due to large pleural effusion. The patient presented with increasing dyspnoea and bloodstained sputum. There is generalised mucosal swelling, reddening and increased vascularity due to chronic bronchitis. Most of the increased secretion has been removed. The extensive effusion has compressed and distorted the bronchi: the right main lumen is more arch-shaped than circular. The posterior wall has been thrust forward and the distal branching is obscured by lateral compression. There was a small peripheral tumour in the right lower lobe, only visible radiographically, and adenocarcinoma cells were found in the pleural fluid.

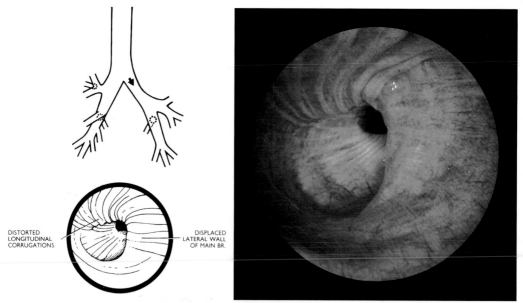

Plate 116

Compression by pleural effusion. Left main bronchus. Left pleuritic pain, with subsequent dyspnoea and night sweats were this patient's complaints. The bronchial tree proved entirely normal, apart from the distortion due to a large pleural effusion. The lateral bronchial wall is markedly displaced medially, distorting the longitudinal corrugations and partially obscuring the bifurcation into upper and lower bronchi, which should clearly be seen from this viewpoint. There was no rigidity of the bronchial tree, in contradistinction to that found when carcinomatous involvement of lymph nodes gives similar distortion. Pleural biopsy: caseating tuberculosis.

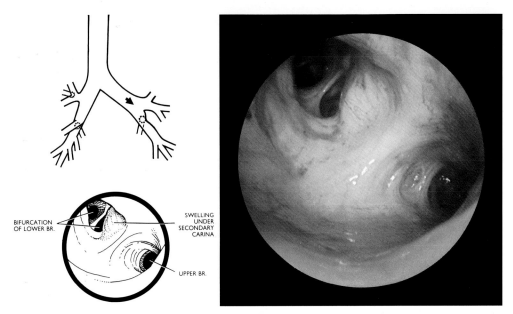

Plate 117

Distortion by enlarged lymph nodes. Division of left main bronchus. Increasing lassitude and pleuritic type pain in the left shoulder, for a few weeks only, drove this patient to her doctor. Radiography revealed partial left upper lobe collapse. Bronchoscopy showed a metastatic deposit in the medial wall of the left main bronchus, a rigid left bronchial tree, tumour tissue in the depths of the left upper bronchus and the distortion shown here due to node involvement under the secondary carina. Biopsy: oat-cell carcinoma. (Compare Plate 148.)

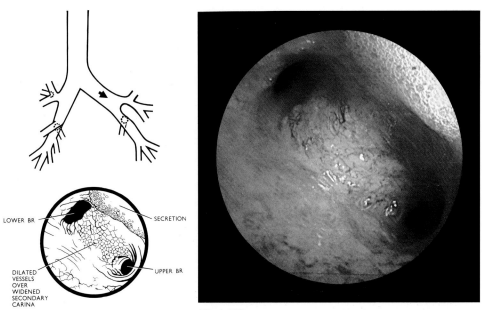

Plate 118

Widening of secondary carina. Division of left main bronchus. The lymph nodes beneath the secondary carina are involved in metastases from bronchial carcinoma. The carina is grossly widened and saddle-shaped: the overlying swollen and irregular mucosa contains a network of dilated vessels. Biopsy proved that it was already invaded by squamous-cell carcinoma. Both upper and lower bronchi are narrowed by the distortion. The generalised reddening and swelling of the mucosa, and excess secretion, were compatible with the long previous history of chronic bronchitis. Recently the cough had become much more irritating and persistent.

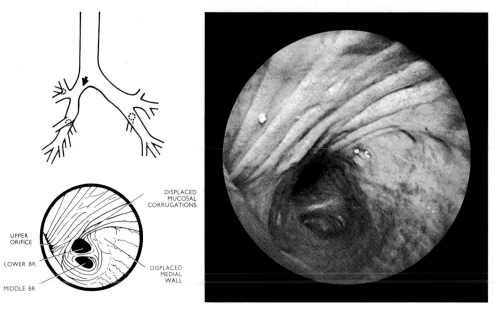

Plate 119

Compression by enlarged lymph nodes. Right main bronchus. A squamous-cell carcinoma of the left lower bronchus has metastasised extensively to the mediastinal lymph nodes. The carina was grossly widened and both main bronchi were compressed. Here the medial wall of the right main bronchus, with its overlying distorted and swollen mucosa, is seen thrust laterally. The posterior wall is pushed forward at the orifice of the upper bronchus by more peripheral node enlargement. The displacement of the prominent mucosal corrugations makes the distortion all the clearer.

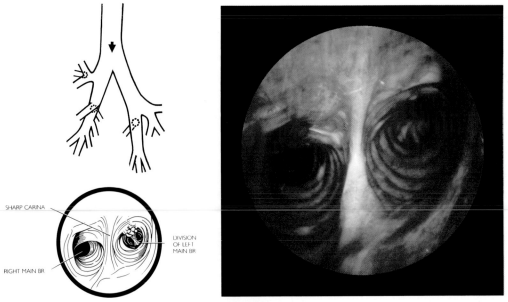

Plate 120

Bronchial displacement due to bilateral lobar collapse. This patient gave a history of recurrent haemoptysis over the previous year. She had no memory of previous respiratory illness. There is a remarkably clear view down both main bronchi from a point in the lower trachea. The carina is exceptionally sharp. The mucosa shews generalised inflammatory changes after removal of bilateral purulent secretions. The findings were due to bilateral lower lobe collapse, associated with bronchiectasis, leading to medial displacement of both main bronchi. (Compare Plates 121, 122 & 130.)

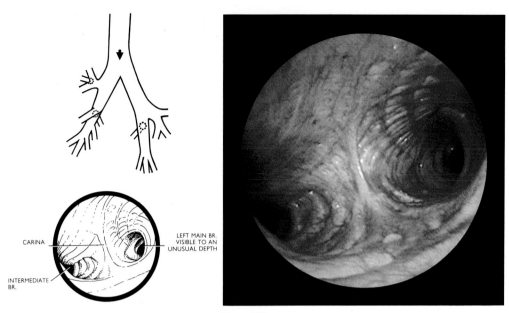

Plate 121

Bronchial displacement due to lobar collapse. Main bifurcation. Most unusual is the ability to see, from this point in the trachea, straight down the left main bronchus to its bifurcation in the distance. This is due to complete collapse of the left lower lobe, with associated bronchiectasis, following tuberculous lobar pneumonia 10 years previously. Consequently there has been medial displacement of the left bronchial tree. The longitudinal corrugations, and particularly the transverse muscle bands, are well seen in the left main bronchus. There is generalised reddening of the mucosa and some increase in secretion associated with the bronchiectasis. The carina and right main bronchus are normal. (Compare Plates 120, 122 & 130.)

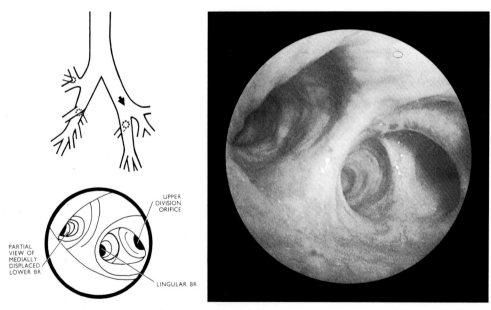

Plate 122

Bronchial displacement due to pulmonary collapse. Division of left main bronchus. In this case it was possible to see a considerable distance down both main bronchi, from the same point proximal to the carina, due to left lower lobe collapse and the consequent medial displacement of the main bronchus. (Compare Plates 120, 121 & 130.) The associated downward swing of the left upper bronchus is very evident as the division of the left main bronchus is approached, as seen here. The upper bronchus forms a direct continuation of the main bronchus and its division is clearly seen, giving the view usually obtained only with the lateral-viewing telescope or fibrescope. (Normally, in some cases only, the lingular bronchus can be seen in this way.)

109

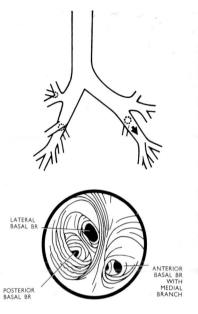

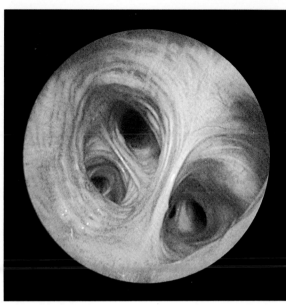

LATERAL
BASAL BR

POSTERIOR
BASAL BR

ANTERIOR
BASAL BR
WITH
MEDIAL
BRANCH

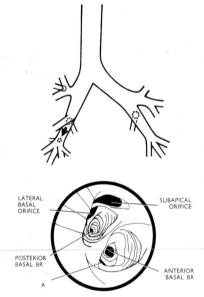

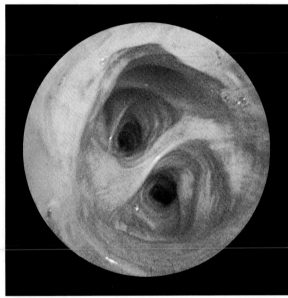

LATERAL
BASAL
ORIFICE

SUBAPICAL
ORIFICE

POSTERIOR
BASAL BR

ANTERIOR
BASAL BR

A

Plates 123 & 124

Bilateral basal bronchiectasis. Basal bronchi. On the left (Plate 123) no significant infection was present and the minimal secretion has been removed. The submucosa is rather atrophic. Most striking is the 'crowding' of the basal bronchi; all can be seen into for an unusual depth from the same vantage point. It is not possible to be dogmatic in naming the orifices because of the distortion, but probably there has been anticlockwise rotation and the likely position is that depicted. On the right (Plate 124) there was considerable mucopuru-lent secretion: this has been removed revealing reddened and slightly swollen mucosa. As on the left, there is some bronchial 'crowding' but, in addition, the anatomical arrangement is not the prevailing pattern. The missing medial basal bronchus is probably replaced by branches from the subapical bronchus and from the unusually large anterior basal bronchus: the orifice of one early branch can be seen at A. (Compare Plates 63, 64 & 125.)

110

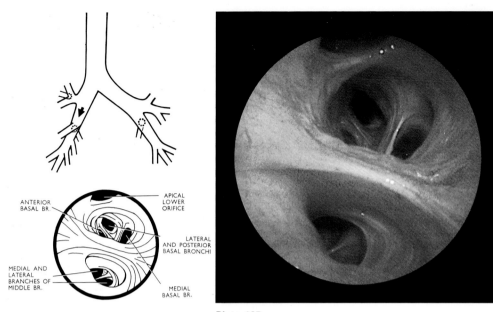

Plate 125

Bronchiectasis. Right middle bronchus. The obliquity of the middle bronchus usually prevents a clear view into it with the forward-viewing rigid telescope but occasionally its division into medial and lateral branches can be seen if the head is turned well to the left and the proximal end of the bronchoscope is lowered as far as possible. Here this view is obtained easily without such manoeuvring, while still retaining the apical lower and basal orifices in the field of vision. This is quite unusual and is due to the middle lobe collapse and downward swing of the middle bronchus. Bronchography revealed extensive bronchiectasis of the middle bronchial branches. Minimal secretion was present and the mucosa was only a little reddened. (Compare Plates 123 & 124.)

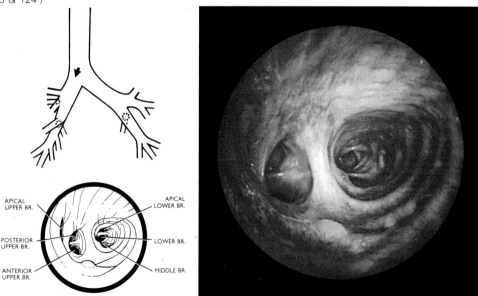

Plate 126

Bronchial displacement due to emphysematous bulla. Right main bronchus. A very large apical bulla was present. In consequence the right upper lobe was compressed downward, swinging the upper bronchus downward with it. The axis of this bronchus is thus no longer at a right angle to the main bronchus, but passes obliquely downward and laterally, making the orifices of its three branches abnormally visible. Both the anterior and posterior orifices are seen clearly with the forward-viewing telescope directed down the main bronchus. The apical orifice could also be inspected unusually easily. The mucosa is reddened with some secretion present. (Compare Plates 127 & 129.) This case also illustrates an example of partial separation of the apical segmental branch of the upper bronchus. (Compare Plates 36 to 38.)

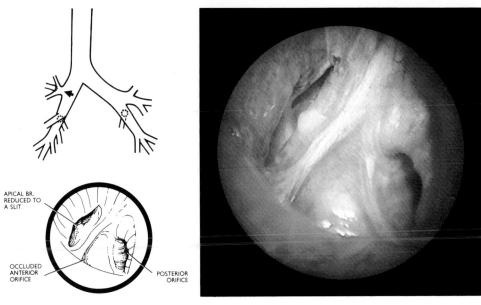

Plate 127

Bronchial displacement due to emphysematous bulla. Right upper bronchus. Lateral-viewing telescope. A large apical bulla has compressed the upper bronchial tree. In this view the effect on the segmental branches of the upper bronchus can be seen: they are all reduced to slitlike orifices. There is some mucosal reddening and a slight increase in secretion.

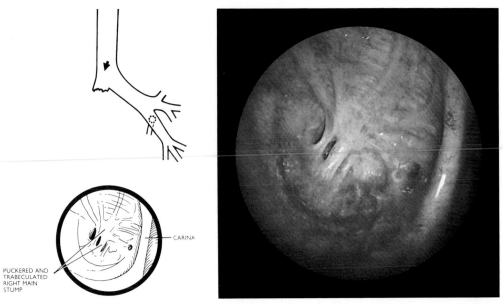

Plate 128

Pneumonectomy for carcinoma. Right main bronchial stump. The carina and a small part of the left main bronchus are on the right of the picture. The puckered and dimpled mucosa, with string-like adhesions overlying the suture lines, fills most of the picture. The operation had been performed four years previously with no sign of recurrence of the squamous-cell carcinoma. (Compare Plates 129, 230 & 231.)

112

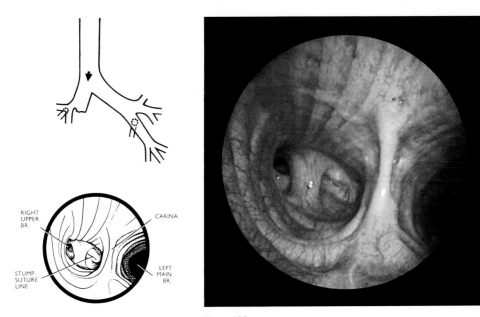

Plate 129

Lobectomy for squamous-cell carcinoma. Carina and right main bronchus. Both the right middle and lower lobes were removed four years previously. The suture line is firm and healthy. Some bronchitic changes are present, including a dilated mucous duct, beside the carina, and generalised mucosal reddening. Following the lobectomy the right upper lobe has expanded to fill the resulting space. In consequence the upper bronchus is displaced downward allowing a view of the anterior and posterior bronchial orifices from the lower trachea. (Compare Plate 126.)

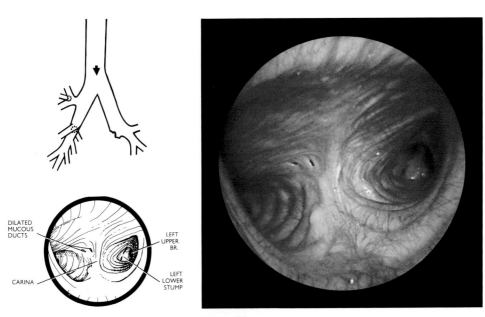

Plate 130

Lobectomy for squamous-cell carinoma. Main bifurcation. A left lower lobectomy had been performed seven years previously. Recent haemoptysis led to bronchoscopy and the discovery of a partially extruded suture, which was removed uneventfully. (Compare Plate 234.) The unusual view of the left upper bronchus and stump, from a point above the carina, is due to the medial and downward displacement of the upper lobe to fill the lobectomy space. (Compare Plate 121.) Bronchitic changes are present, including dilated mucous ducts to the right of the carina. (Compare Plates 58 & 181.)

113

CHAPTER 8

TUMOURS

At bronchoscopy, it is the way that a tumour has behaved anatomically, rather than its histological type, that is of importance. Distortion or invasion of the visible bronchi and appreciable involvement of local lymph nodes will have an immediate impact on the bronchoscopic findings; the degree of malignancy, as shown histologically, will only have significance later in relation to treatment and prognosis. Although squamous-cell tumours tend to superficial necrosis, and oat-cell to early spread to lymph nodes, it is impossible in the majority of cases to predict the histology, for tumours of widely different types may give remarkably similar endoscopic pictures (Plates 133, 153, 158, 160 & 175). An occasional exception is the carcinoid adenoma which, characteristically, presents as a very red tumour somewhat reminiscent of a cherry or mulberry (Plate 169).

Bronchoscopically, tumours, or metastatic lymph node enlargements therefrom, may produce visible changes of three main types: (1) simple distortion of the normal anatomy by external pressure on the bronchial tree, (2) involvement of the bronchial wall with local distortion or ulceration of the mucosa, (3) intraluminal eruption of the growth.

Simple distortion of the bronchial tree has been described in Chapter 7. It is commonly due to secondary lymph node enlargement; thus, widening of the adjacent secondary carina frequently accompanies other evidence of bronchial tumours. Widening of the main carina, bulging of the medial walls of the main bronchi, or distortion of the trachea by enlarged subcarinal or paratracheal nodes are clear bronchoscopic signs of inoperability. Such swellings often lead to nodular distortion of the trachea, carina or main bronchi and ultimate ulceration and fungation of the growth into the tracheal or bronchial lumina (Plates 134 to 141). Distortion and/or obliteration of the longitudinal mucosal corrugations are common features emphasising this picture (Plates 102, 136 & 140; see also Chapter 7). Primary carcinoma of the trachea is extremely rare (Plates 131 to 133). The mucosa overlying nodes involved in tumour is frequently vascular and inflamed (Plates 113 & 118), but the degree of malignant involvement may be much more advanced than suspected visually (Plate 142).

Submucosal mural growths, often encircling or partly encircling the lumen and greatly reducing or closing it, are common (Plates 145 to 149 & 161). The narrowing may be uniform or irregular. The mucosa can be pale, yellow and slightly raised, with a clear, delineated edge indicating the visible limit of the creeping tumour (Plates 144 to 146), or it may closely imitate simple inflammation, with swelling and reddening only (Ch. 6). Nevertheless, tissues involved by growth tend to be more rigid and, indeed, are often firmly fixed in position, which must immediately suggest extensive tumour involvement (Plates 149 & 151). It should be remembered, however, that tuberculosis, radiotherapy and sarcoidosis can also produce rigidity. Frequently, particularly in more advanced growths, this is a prominent finding sometimes preventing further passage of the rigid bronchoscope even in the main bronchi (Plate 151). A less advanced mural growth may present as a local tumour formation narrowing the lumen, with reddening and telangiectasia of the overlying mucosa: elevation, deviation or cessation of the longitudinal mucosal corrugations are common findings in such cases (Plates 145 & 147). Similarly a mural growth in a large bronchus can obscure the characteristic curved ridging due to the bronchial cartilages (Plate 151). A mucosal biopsy, taken from an apparently inflamed area proximal to a tumour, not infrequently confirms malignant spread beyond that which was clearly visible bronchoscopically. In cases of carcinomatous lymphangitis, the bronchial mucosa may be widely involved and yield positive results from multiple biopsies (Plates 142 & 143). Tuberculosis and sarcoidosis can produce a very similar miliary picture (Plates 82 & 206).

An intraluminal growth may prove to be the primary itself; an extension from the primary; or rupture of a secondary lymph node deposit through the bronchial wall. This differentiation may be impossible to make bronchoscopically, but extremes in this range of possibilities can usually be appreciated: a small benign papillomatous endobronchial growth may be removed completely at endoscopy leaving a bronchial tree otherwise entirely normal (Plate 172); on the other hand, marked carinal blunting, subcarinal widening, or tracheal compression, with growth erupting through the carina and possibly tracheal wall, carries its own sinister indication of adjacent, extensive lymph node involvement (Plates 134 to 138). A similar situation may evolve from enlarged nodes posterior to the main bronchi (Plate 140).

Most intraluminal tumours seen endoscopically, however, fall into an intermediate category, presenting as a projection of irregular abnormal tissue replacing the mucosa. The extent of the growth varies from a localised surface abnormality (Plates 150 & 170) to a mass of tissue that widely involves the bronchial wall (Plates 151 to 154). This tissue may partially or completely occlude the bronchial lumen (Plates 153, 157, 160, 162 & 163); it may be fleshy and lobulated (Plates 153 & 168), glistening and tongue-like (Plate 165) or, very commonly, necrotic and white or cream-coloured (Plates 158, 159, 187, 191 & 195). Blood streaking and engorged vessels are often present on the surface (Plates 153 to 157, 166, 168 & 169). In larger bronchi tumours are often seen before they obstruct the airway completely, but smaller visible bronchi frequently have their lumina obviously closed by growth at the time of bronchoscopy: a small portion of growth protruding from an obviously blocked or very greatly reduced, segmental orifice is a common sight (Plates 162 to 164, 166, 168 & 169). Cases showing a variety of features are also common (Plate 182).

A type of tumour worth particular mention is that which grows intrabronchially, in peduncular fashion, to present to the bronchoscopist much more proximally than its point of origin (Plates 159, 165, 166, 169 & 175). This situation is discussed further in Chapter 9.

The great majority of visible tumours prove to be bronchial carcinomata: occasional, usually red, carcinoid tumours (adenomata) which bleed readily, will be seen (Plates 169 & 170), but others are rare. Metastases, from primary tumours elsewhere, although commonly revealed radiographically in the pulmonary parenchyma, are most unusual in the bronchial tree (Plates 174 & 175). Benign tumours usually have a healthy covering mucosa (Plates 171 to 173): chondromata present a particularly smooth, pale surface and hard consistency (Plates 176 & 177). Whatever their histological type, tumours commonly produce bronchial obstruction and hence retained secretion and infection: carcinoma is a common cause of lung abscess in cigarette-smoking communities. As mentioned in Chapter 6, the local inflammatory reaction produced by a tumour, even if bronchial obstruction is not marked, may closely imitate simple inflammation if the tumour itself is not visible (Plate 67). A foreign body may also be obscured by the reaction it produces and can easily be mistaken for a carcinoma unless delicate feeling with the forceps is undertaken routinely in all suspicious cases (Ch. 10).

It should be appreciated that in a large proportion of cases the secondary inflammatory reaction and partial obstruction produced by a tumour lead to sufficient pus formation to obscure vision in its vicinity. This must be removed before the true situation can be appreciated, but the greatest care is needed to avoid trauma to the tumour or surrounding mucosa when using the sucker. It is characteristic of some tumours that the slightest trauma can produce brisk haemorrhage which obscures the field as completely as did the pus that was removed. Great gentleness, without haste, is thus at a premium if successful diagnosis is to be achieved (Ch. 9).

Finally it must be stressed how important it is to explore the bronchial tree systematically and as thoroughly as possible; a tumour can readily be missed if this is not done (Plates 179, 180, 181 & 182).

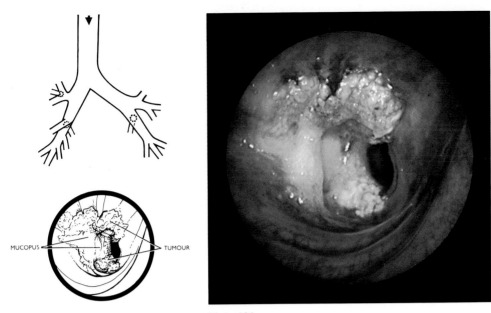

Plate 131

Carcinoma. Trachea. This is an example of the rarely occurring, primary tracheal tumour. It is seen to have crept round a considerable part of the tracheal circumference. There is copious purulent material present and a little spontaneous bleeding. The patient presented with a history of multiple pulmonary infections with no obvious cause: presumably aspiration phenomena from the infected tumour tissue. There was also weakness, weight loss, cough and a recent small haemoptysis. Biopsy: poorly differentiated squamous-cell carcinoma. Radiotherapy gave considerable temporary relief. (Compare Plates 132, 133, 174 & 211.)

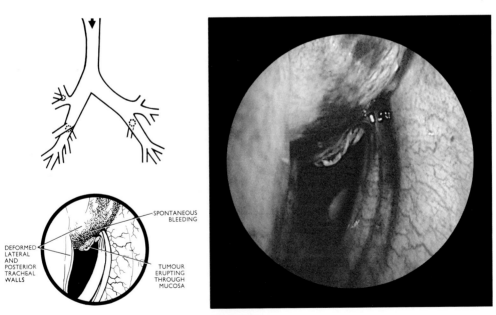

Plate 132

Carcinoma. Trachea. Bronchoscopy was undertaken for persistent haemoptysis: the bleeding tumour erupting through the posterior tracheal wall is the obvious cause. Radiotherapy had been given to this area seven years previously for a malignant thymoma. The resulting rigid distortion of the right lateral and posterior tracheal walls is well seen. The tumour responded to further radiation and the haemoptysis was controlled. Biopsy: squamous-cell carcinoma, with no sign of recurrent thymoma. Primary carcinoma of the trachea is extremely rare: this one may well have been radiation-induced by the first course of treatment. (Compare Plates 131, 133, 174 & 211.)

117

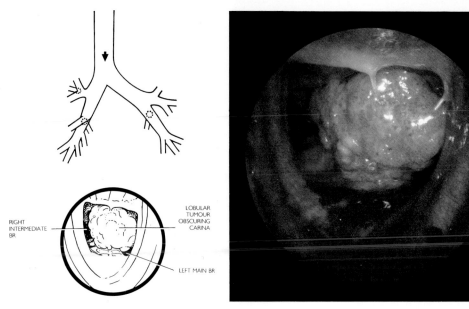

Plate 133

Carcinoma. Trachea. This heavily-smoking, elderly patient had remained remarkably fit throughout his life. He presented with only a three month history of cough, yellow sputum and a recent small haemoptysis. A large, lobulated, fleshy tumour is seen arising from the posterior wall of the lower trachea. The carina and left main bronchus are obscured; the lumen of the right main bronchus greatly reduced. The mucosa is reddened and there is an increase in secretion. Minimal sucker trauma is seen on the anterior tracheal wall. Biopsy: squamous-cell carcinoma. (Compare Plates 131, 132, 174 & 211.)

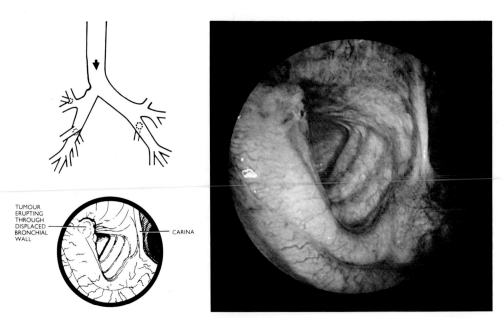

Plate 134

Carcinoma of trachea. Main bifurcation. In the lower trachea, from its right lateral wall, a mass projects into the lumen. Tumour is breaking through the posterior portion of the mass where the surface is distorted and nodular. Biopsy: squamous-cell carcinoma. This tracheal lesion was produced by direct spread from a large right paratracheal lymph node involved in metastic deposition of cancer from a primary site in the posterior segmental branch of the right upper bronchus. (Compare Plate 93.)

118

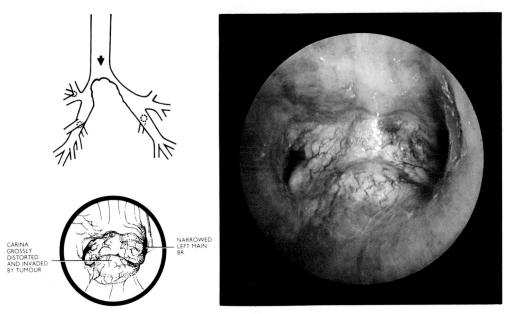

Plate 135

Carcinoma. Carina and main bronchi. This is a late stage of subcarinal lymph node invasion by metastatic tumour. A right middle lobectomy had been performed for carcinoma six months previously. The main clinical finding was loud, persistent wheezing over the left upper, anterior chest. The carina itself is invaded and cancer is erupting through the mucosa over a wide area. The central lymph node mass has narrowed both main bronchi by displacing their medial walls laterally. These walls were invaded and destroyed over a considerable length. The surrounding mucosa is reddened and swollen due to associated inflammatory reaction and probably some cancerous invasion. Biopsy: adenocarcinoma.

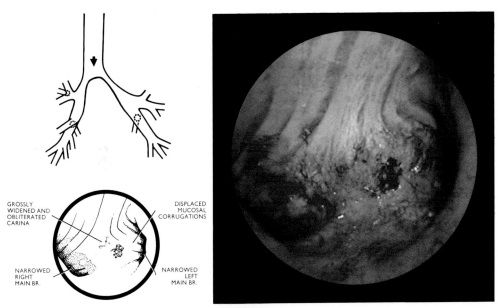

Plate 136

Carcinoma. Carina and main bronchi. An advanced stage of subcarinal lymph node invasion by bronchial carcinoma is seen here. The patient presented with persistent, stridulous wheezing, cough and dyspnoea of recent onset. Superior vena caval obstruction was present. The carina and subcarinal areas are grossly widened so that both main bronchi are reduced to slits. The overlying mucosa is reddened and invaded by tumour tissue. The displacement of the longitudinal corrugations emphasises the distortion. Biopsy: polygonal-cell carcinoma.

119

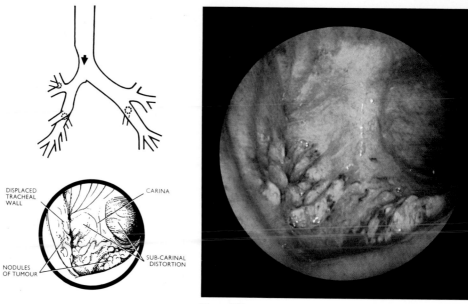

Plate 137

Extensive carcinoma. Main bifurcation. The carinal edge is still clearly visible, but the subcarinal area is widened. This is particularly noticeable on the right, where the distortion of the lower tracheal wall by paratracheal lymph node enlargement has also added to the marked reduction of the bronchial lumen. Multiple tumour deposits are seen overlying the distorted areas. The full length of the right main bronchus was similarly involved and rigid. The location of the primary tumour was uncertain. Biopsy, undifferentiated carcinoma. (Compare Plates 51, 138, 205 & 207.)

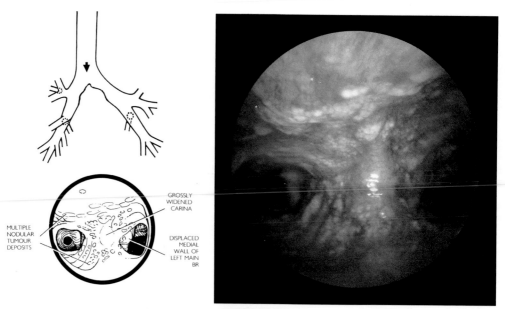

Plate 138

Carcinoma. Main bifurcation. This patient presented with a five month history of increasing lethargy and dyspnoea, with additional dry cough for five weeks. Chest radiography revealed bilateral scattered shadowing. The subcarinal area is a little widened, protrusion of the medial bronchial wall being most obvious in the left main bronchus. The mucosa is reddened and contains nodules diffusely scattered in the carinal area, lower trachea and both main bronchi. There is also some increase in secretion, seen on the posterior tracheal wall. These findings suggested the possibility of sarcoidosis, for no primary tumour was found in the thorax or elsewhere. Biopsy: poorly-differentiated squamous-cell carcinoma. (Compare Plates 51, 137, 205 & 207.)

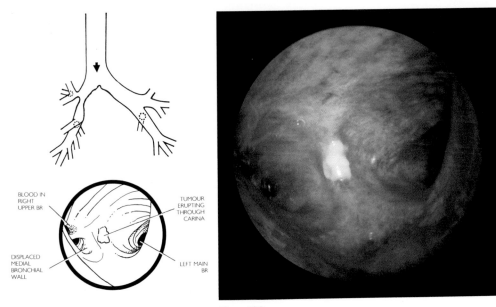

Plate 139

Carcinoma. Carina and main bronchi. There is widespread reddening and swelling of the mucosa. Considerable excess secretion has been removed; minimal sucker trauma is evident. The left main bronchus is otherwise normal. Although there is no proximal subcarinal widening, there is an unusual deposit of white tumour tissue on the carinal edge. The right intermediate bronchus is almost occluded by displacement of its medial wall, presumably by mediastinal lymph node enlargement. Extensive bleeding tumour tissue involves the lateral wall of the intermediate bronchus and, in the far left of the picture, is seen to occlude the upper bronchus. The extent of tumour invasion obscures the primary source. Biopsy: oat-cell carcinoma.

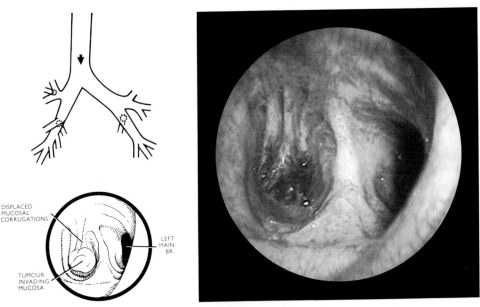

Plate 140

Carcinoma. Carina and main bronchi. The patient presented with increased cough and persistent wheeze. Lymph nodes, invaded by tumour, have displaced forward the posterior wall of the right main bronchus, thus almost obliterating the lumen. The distorted, prominent, mucosal corrugations makes this very clear. At the point of maximal displacement, tumour has invaded the mucosa and spontaneous bleeding has occurred. The carina is not widened but there is slight displacement. The right upper orifice is obscured by the distortion. Mild, generalised, bronchitic changes are present in the mucosa. Biopsy: poorly differentiated squamous-cell carcinoma. (Compare Plates 109 & 110.)

121

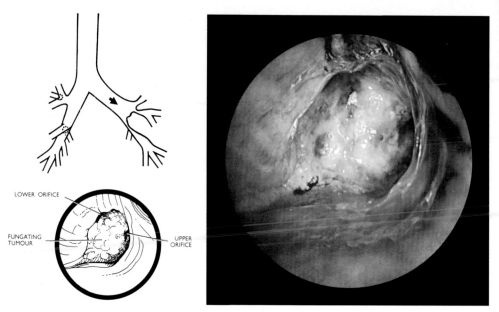

Plate 141

Fungating carcinoma. Bifurcation of left main bronchus. The presenting symptom was a history of rapid onset dyspnoea two months previously. This was followed by recent left pleuritic pain and, finally, a small hae-moptysis. Already the tumour is very extensive and necrotic. It is seen as a fungating mass erupting from the lymph nodes beneath the secondary carina between upper and lower bronchi. The upper bronchus was com-pletely obstructed by the primary tumour and the lower considerably reduced in calibre: clearly the cause of the dyspnoea. Biopsy: poorly differentiated squamous-cell carcinoma.

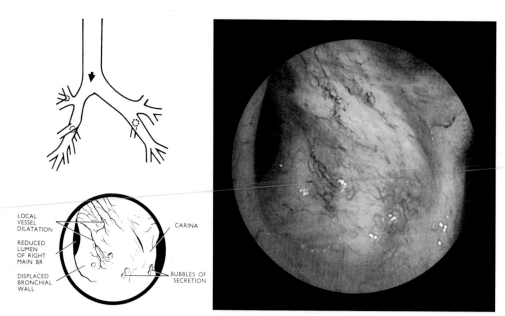

Plate 142

Local mucosal vessel dilatation overlying cancerous lymph node. Right main bronchus. The carina, still with a sharp edge, is seen to the right of the picture. There is, however, marked subcarinal lymph node enlargement due to secondary deposition of carcinoma. This has thrust the medial wall of the right main bronchus into its lumen, obliterating the cartilage outlines. Over the swelling the mucosal vessels have become prominently dilated; an unusual finding in the case of benign swellings. Isolated local vascularity should always rouse suspicions of an underlying pathological process, but may sometimes occur for no apparent reason. Biopsy: undifferentiated carcinoma with lymphatic invasion. (Compare Plate 53.)

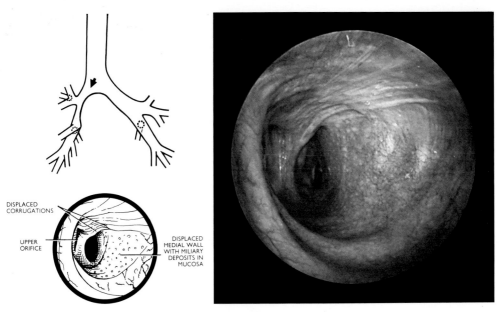

Plate 143

Carcinoma. Miliary deposition. Right main bronchus. The medial bronchial wall has been displaced so far laterally, by mediastinal lymph node enlargement, that the lumen of the intermediate bronchus has been reduced to a narrow oval. Over the surface of this swelling can be seen the faint outlines of pale miliary deposits. The patient had extensive metastatic involvement of bone and was becoming increasingly dyspnoeic from widespread invasion of the pulmonary lymphatics. Mucosal biopsy: miliary deposits of poorly differentiated squamous-cell carcinoma with extensive invasion of lymphatics. (Compare Plates 82 & 206.)

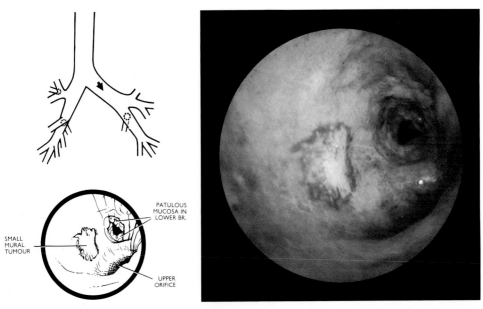

Plate 144

Carcinoma. Left main bronchus. The bifurcation into upper and lower bronchi is well seen on the right of the picture. Bronchitis was present, accounting for the mucosal irregularity in the lower bronchus. The main feature is the small, raised, irregular area on the medial wall of the main bronchus. This was thought to be a secondary deposit, from a pre-existing right-sided squamous-cell carcinoma, but a generous biopsy revealed unequivocal adenocarcinoma. (Compare Plates 179 & 180.)

123

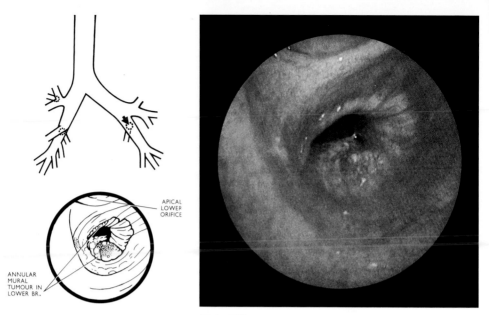

Plate 145

Carcinoma. Left lower bronchus. Bronchoscopy followed the discovery of carcinoma cells in the sputum. The mucosa is generally reddened. At the periphary can be seen the inferior margin of the apical lower bronchial orifice. Beyond this a tumour has involved the bronchial wall, spreading in annular fashion, to raise the longitudinal elastic bundles into prominence. The macroscopic proximal edge of the tumour is thus clearly delineated. The point of maximum growth is seen anteriorly; here a little blood and a yellow nodule indicate an early breach in the mucosa. Although diminished by the rigid ring of tumour, the lumen is still very adequate: hence the lack of radiological change. Biopsy: squamous-cell carcinoma. (Compare Plates 146 & 149.)

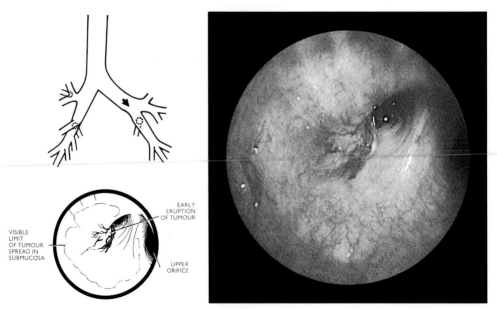

Plate 146

Carcinoma. Left main bronchus. The mucosa is generally reddened and throws into contrast the yellow colouration of the area involved with tumour. This has erupted through the mucosa on the medial wall of the left main bronchus and here there is a marked increase in vascularity. Biopsy: squamous-cell carcinoma. (Compare Plates 145 & 149.)

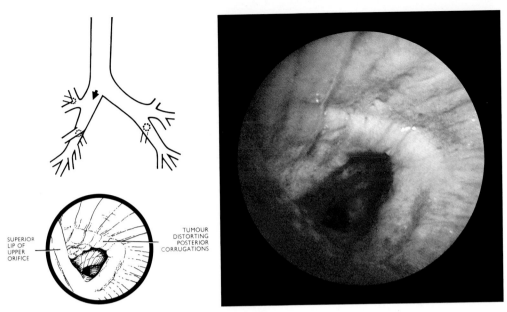

Plate 147

Carcinoma. Right main bronchus. The primary tumour was in the right upper bronchus. There has been sub-mucosal spread from the orifice of the right upper bronchus, obliquely across the posterior wall of the main bronchus to involve its medial wall also. This situation can sometimes suggest anatomical anomalies. (Compare Plate 52.)

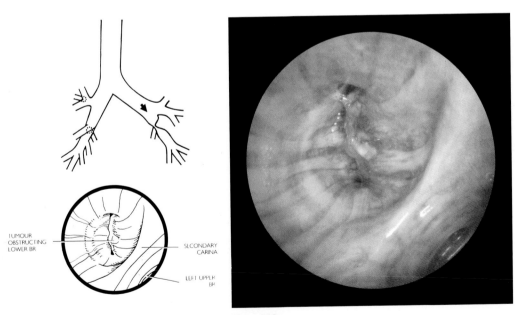

Plate 148

Carcinoma. Left lower bronchus. This elderly smoker had suffered an influenza-like illness three months previously which had left him with a persistant cough and sputum. Chest radiography revealed a mass in the apical segment of the left lower lobe: presumed to be a primary carcinoma. The lower bronchus is almost occluded by a large swelling of the lateral wall: its surface is irregular and nodular, indicating early tumour eruption into the lumen. Whether this swelling is local node involvement or direct spread from the primary tumour in the apical lower segment is uncertain. Biopsy: squamous-cell carcinoma. (Compare Plate 117.)

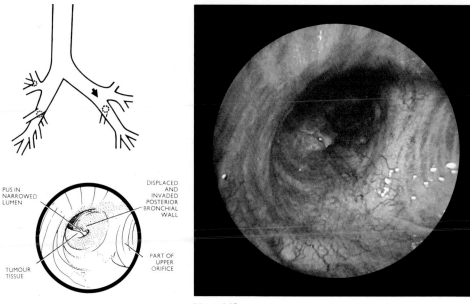

Plate 149

Carcinoma. Left lower bronchus. Here, as in Plates 145 & 146, but at a later stage, a carcinoma has involved, in annular fashion, the wall of the lower bronchus. There was great rigidity in this region, easily detected with the rigid bronchoscope. There is marked local inflammatory reaction, with pus present. The lumen has been considerably reduced and finally blocked by pus. Cough, haemoptysis and a deflated lower lobe led to the bronchoscopy. Biopsy: oat-cell carcinoma.

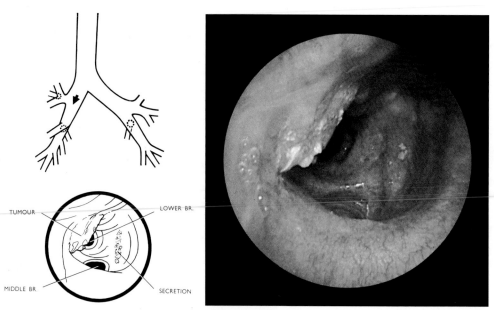

Plate 150

Carcinoma. Right main bronchus. On the lateral bronchial wall, a little beyond the upper orifice, is an irregular tumour protruding into the lumen. The mucosa has been breached and necrotic areas are visible on the surface. The mucosa elsewhere is only a little reddened with slight prominence of the vessels. Some secretion is present on the medial bronchial wall and beyond this can be seen the division into middle and lower bronchi. Biopsy: well differentiated squamous-cell carcinoma. Subsequent successful removal and histological examination showed this to be a locally invasive primary tumour. A persistent increase in this patient's cough had been disregarded: only following a small haemoptysis was he referred for investigation. The chest radiograph was normal.

126

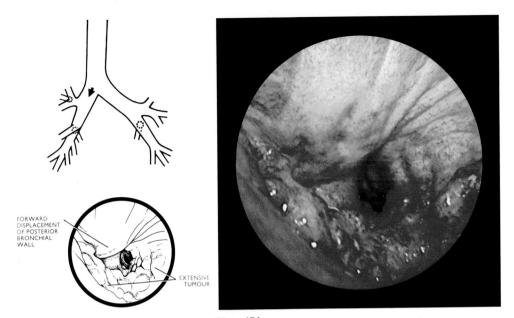

Plate 151

Carcinoma. Right main bronchus. Extensive, fleshy, tumour tissue has involved the medial, anterior and lateral walls of the main bronchus just proximal to the upper orifice. The longitudinal corrugations are clearly distorted. The tissues were rigid in this area and the protruding, posterior bronchial wall was unaffected by pulmonary inflation: signs indicating that spread to local lymph nodes has already occurred. Biopsy: undifferentiated carcinoma. (Compare Plate 81.)

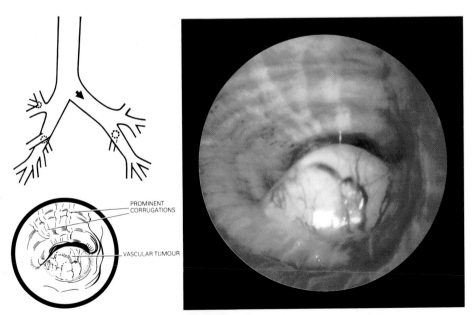

Plate 152

Carcinoma. Left main bronchus. This 72-year-old lady gave up her heavy smoking three months previously when she suddenly became hoarse. Her chronic cough and dyspnoea also worsened. There is generalised reddening and swelling of the mucosa with prominent longitudinal corrugations. A large tumour mass is seen on the anterior wall of the left main bronchus with dilated vessels on its surface. The left vocal cord was paralysed. Biopsy: squamous cell carcinoma. (Compare Plates 8, 98 & 163.)

127

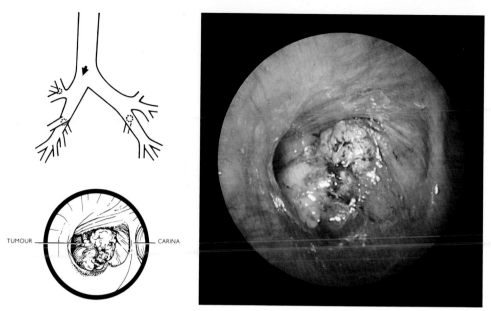

Plate 153

Carcinoma. Right main bronchus. This bronchoscopy was undertaken because the patient presented with a myasthenic syndrome involving proximal limb muscles. A large, lobulated, fleshy mass is seen, greatly reducing the right main bronchial lumen. This was considered to be a primary tumour, originating in the right main bronchial wall close to the carina, rather than an intraluminal eruption of a cancerous subcarinal node: no growth could be found elsewhere in the bronchial tree, either by radiology or bronchoscopy. There is a little spontaneous bleeding on the tumour surface, explaining the more recent additional symptom of minor haemoptysis. Biopsy: oat-cell carcinoma.

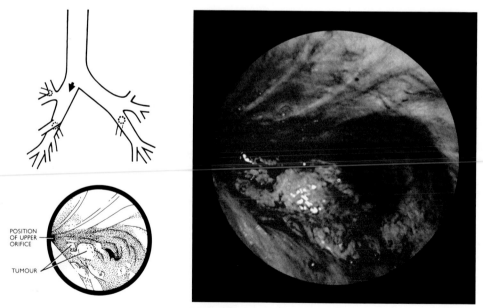

Plate 154

Carcinoma. Right main bronchus. The mucosa shows the usual reddening and swelling due to bronchitis; the longitudinal corrugations are prominent, revealing the position of the right upper orifice. There had been a significant increase in this patient's chronic cough with sputum and persistent haemoptysis. A collapsed right upper lobe was revealed radiologically. On the anterior and lateral bronchial walls is a large, fleshy, vascular tumour which has occluded the upper bronchial orifice. Biopsy: squamous-cell carcinoma.

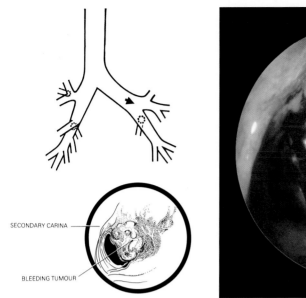

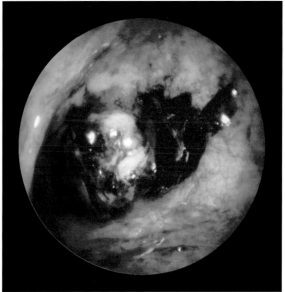

Plate 155

Carcinoma. Left upper bronchus. This patient presented with a left-sided hemiparesis, cough and haemoptysis. Radiography, revealed a rounded shadow in the left upper lung field. The secondary carina between upper and lower bronchi is seen to the far left of the picture. There is a large, bleeding tumour growing down the left upper bronchus and presenting at its orifice. The surrounding mucosa is reddened and swollen. A brain scan revealed a presumed cerebral metastasis. Biopsy: poorly-differentiated squamous cell carcinoma. (Compare Plates 156, 158 & 159.)

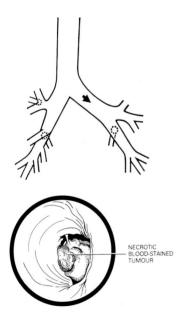

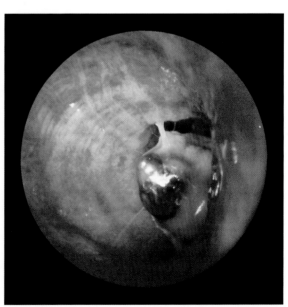

Plate 156

Carcinoma. Left main bronchus. This patient presented with increase in his chronic cough and recurrent, small haemoptyses. The bronchial mucosa is reddened and swollen. Some secretion has already been removed. A necrotic, purulent and blood-stained tumour is erupting from the upper orifice and nearly obstructs the left main bronchus. Biopsy: squamous-cell carcinoma. (Compare Plates 155, 158 & 159.)

129

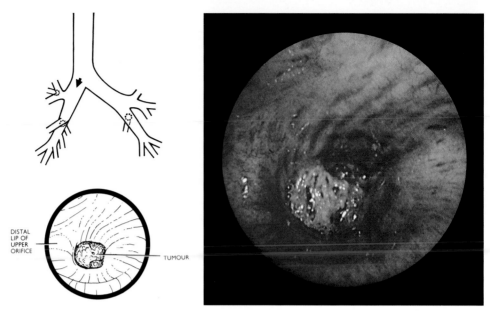

Plate 157

Polypoid carcinoma. Right main bronchus. The patient presented with wheeze, dyspnoea and repeated minor haemoptyses. The radiograph revealed marked overinflation of the right lung, most notable on expiration, due to air trapping. The mucosa is generally reddened and swollen. A large polypoid tumour is seen growing up the intermediate bronchus and largely obstructing the lumen. The tumour surface displays prominent vascularity and there is minor spontaneous bleeding. Biopsy: squamous-cell carcinoma.

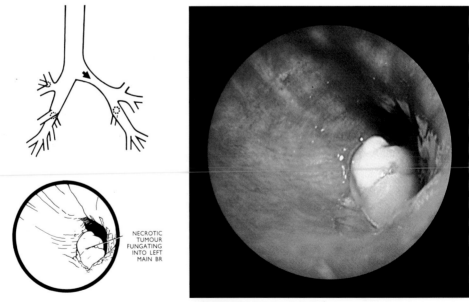

Plate 158

Carcinoma. Left main bronchus. Purulent secretion has already been removed. The mucosa is generally reddened. Mucosal corrugation is seen on the posterior wall and some secretion adheres to the lateral wall. The medial bronchial wall is thrust laterally by lymph nodes enlarged by metastatic carcinoma. Erupting from the upper bronchus, and largely occluding the main bronchial lumen, is a large, yellow, fungating, necrotic tumour. Biopsy: oat-cell carcinoma. (Compare Plates 155, 156 & 159.)

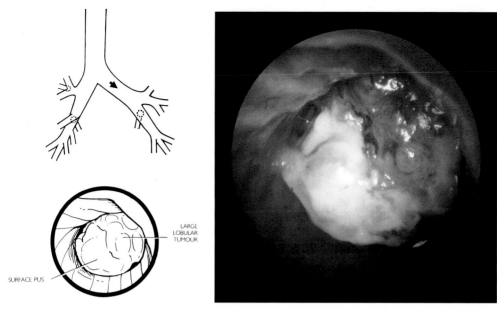

Plate 159

Carcinoma. Left main bronchus. The patient reported intermittent left chest pain, with increasing dyspnoea, for three months and, latterly, episodes of haemoptysis. Chest radiography revealed complete collapse of the left lung. The left main bronchus is occluded by a large, fleshy, lobulated tumour, partly obscured by purulent secretion and blood. The distal origin of this freely movable (i.e. pedunculated) tumour was uncertain because its bloody nature precluded all peripheral exploration or bronchoscopic removal. Biopsy: squamous-cell carcinoma. (Compare Plates 155, 156 & 158.)

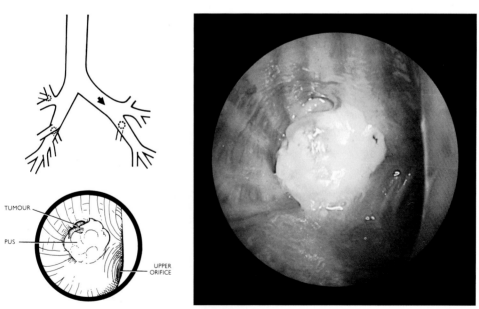

Plate 160

Carcinoma. Left lower bronchus. The patient had already received treatment for a number of infections of the left lower lobe before being referred for bronchoscopy. The orifice of the lower bronchus is completely occluded by a fleshy tumour. There is considerable purulent secretion on its surface but the adjacent mucosa is healthy. A large part of the tumour was removed at rigid bronchoscopy, with the release of a quantity of pus and considerable symptomatic relief for the patient. Biopsy: squamous-cell carcinoma. (Compare Plates 165, 195 & 196.)

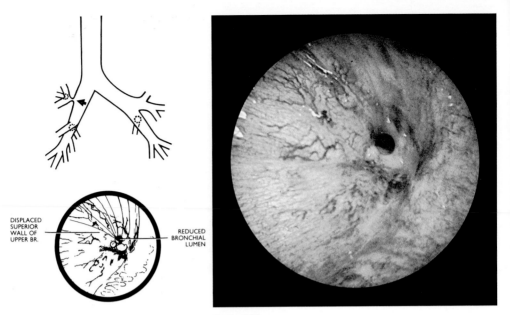

Plate 161

Carcinoma. Right upper orifice. Lateral-viewing telescope. Bronchoscopy was undertaken because of poor response to chemotherapy for proven tuberculosis of the right upper lobe in an elderly, smoking male: a double diagnosis was suspected. No detail of the upper bronchial division and segmental orifices can be made out, for the lumen is largely occluded by tumour invasion of the bronchial wall. Tortuous, engorged vessels run over the tumour surface and minimal spontaneous bleeding is present. Biopsy: squamous-cell carcinoma.

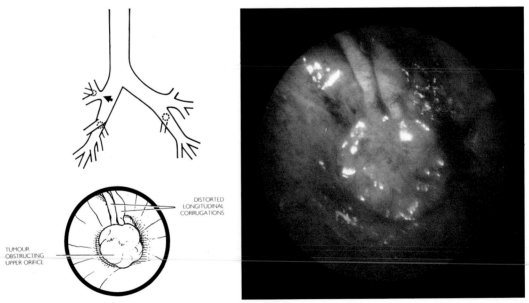

Plate 162

Carcinoma. Right upper bronchus. Lateral-viewing telescope. This chronic bronchitic patient presented with a two-month history of change in his cough habit, increase in dyspnoea, some right upper chest pain and, finally, a small haemoptysis. Chest radiography revealed complete deflation of the right upper lobe. A large, fleshy tumour occludes the bronchial lumen. The surrounding mucosa is reddened and swollen, making the longitudinal corrugations very prominent. There is a little bleeding. Biopsy: squamous-cell carcinoma.

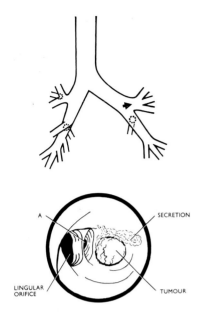

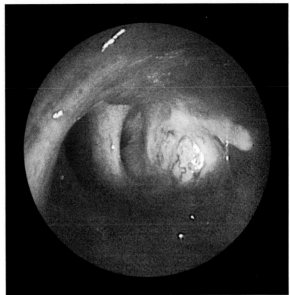

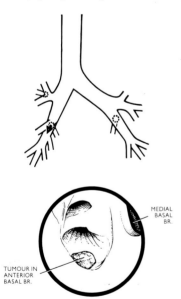

Plate 163

Carcinoma. Left upper orifice. Lateral-viewing telescope. A normal anatomical variation exists in this case: the upper bronchus divides directly into three branches instead of the more usual two. Orifice 'A' probably represents an independent superior branch of the lingular bronchus. The most superior of the three orifices is occluded by a protruding smooth yellow tumour. No biopsy was obtained directly from the tumour (pre-fibrescope era): adjacent mucosal specimens were normal. Metastatic growth had already involved the left recurrent laryngeal nerve, clearly demonstrated at bronchoscopy by left vocal cord paralysis. Understandably, the patient had presented with a hoarse voice. The radiograph revealed collapse of the upper lobe, sparing the lingula, and an enlarged left hilar shadow. (Compare Plates 8, 98 & 152.)

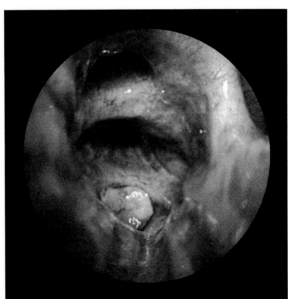

Plate 164

Carcinoma. Right basal system. Pain from hypertrophic pulmonary osteoarthropathy drove this patient to seek advice. Radiography showed the tumour occupying the major part of the anterior basal segment. The usual changes of bronchitis can be seen in this close-up photograph of the basal orifices. A small portion of yellow tumour tissue is protruding from the anterior basal bronchus. This is only part of a large tumour which had grown, in polypoid fashion, up the segmental bronchus to present at its orifice. There was no evidence of spread to intrathoracic lymph nodes so that surgical removal appeared a possibility. Biopsy: poorly differentiated squamous-cell carcinoma.

133

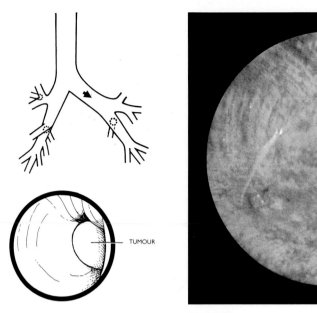

Plate 165

Polypoid carcinoma. Left main bronchus. The patient was elderly with only one minimal symptom; recent on-set of dyspnoea. Complete collapse of the left upper lobe was revealed radiographically. The left main bronchus is almost occluded by a very smooth fleshy, mobile tumour. This was largely removed bronchoscopically, revealing its origin to be the depths of the left upper bronchus and relieving the patient's dyspnoea. Biopsy: oat-cell carcinoma. (Compare Plates 160, 195 & 196.)

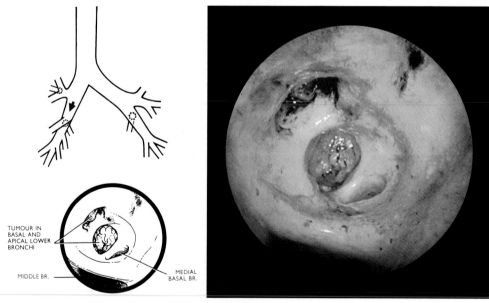

Plate 166

Carcinoma. Right lower bronchus. The patient gave a history of increasing cough for one year and lethargy for some weeks; he had also suffered a small, recent haemoptysis. There was partial collapse of the right lower lobe. Fleshy tumour is clearly seen almost obstructing the basal system beyond the medial basal bronchus. Less obvious, seen obliquely, is bleeding tumour in the apical lower bronchus, presumably the source of the haemoptysis. The radiograph indicated a large mass in the right lower lobe: the common source of the two finger-like projections of the tumour growing up separate bronchi. Biopsy of both: identical squamous-cell carcinoma.

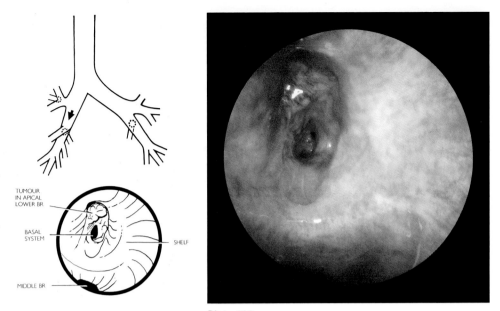

Plate 167

Carcinoma. Right apical lower bronchus. A heavy smoker for 50 years, this bronchitic patient complained of increased productive cough and worsening dyspnoea for 10 weeks only. Chest radiography revealed a large peripheral mass in the apical segment of the right lower lobe. An irregular, lobulated and bloody tumour is seen erupting from the apical lower bronchial orifice. The irregularity of the lateral wall of the lower bronchus indicates spread to this area. The lumen of this bronchus is also narrowed, suggesting pressure from enlarged local lymph nodes. Biopsy: poorly differentiated squamous-cell carcinoma.

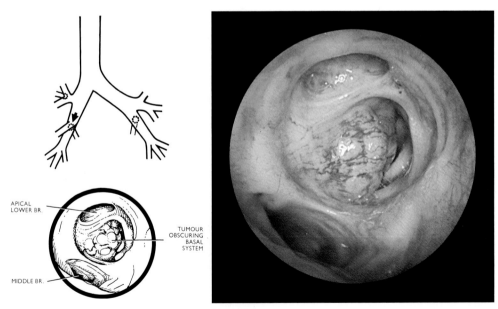

Plate 168

Carcinoma. Right lower bronchus. The only symptom was a few weeks of increasing dyspnoea. This proved to be due to a large right pleural effusion. The presumed primary tumour is seen as a small, lobulated, fleshy mass on the lateral wall of the lower bronchus, arising just beyond the apical lower orifice. Widespread dissemination soon occurred. Biopsy: undifferentiated carcinoma.

135

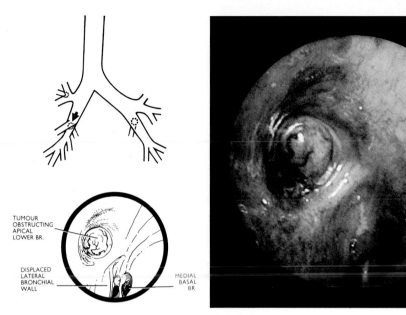

TUMOUR
OBSTRUCTING
APICAL
LOWER BR.

DISPLACED
LATERAL
BRONCHIAL
WALL

MEDIAL
BASAL
BR.

Plate 169

Adenoma. Right lower bronchus. Protruding from the apical lower bronchus is a red, cherry-like tumour. This represents only a small peduncular projection of a much larger tumour beyond vision. Indicative of its presence, however, is the medial displacement of the lateral bronchial wall, reducing the lumen to about half normal. Biopsy: carcinoid adenoma. Successful surgical removal was achieved by lower lobectomy. (See also Plate 233.)

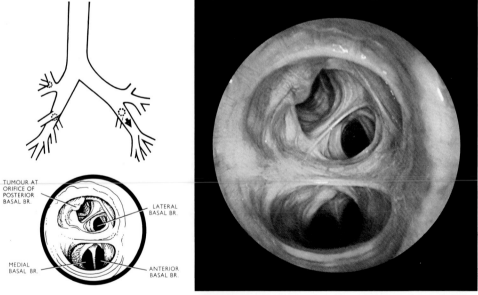

TUMOUR AT
ORIFICE OF
POSTERIOR
BASAL BR.

LATERAL
BASAL BR.

MEDIAL
BASAL BR.

ANTERIOR
BASAL BR.

Plate 170

Adenoma. Left basal system. The anatomy of the basal branching is very clearly seen in this photograph. (Compare Plate 33.) The patient was an extremely fit nonsmoker; hence the clean mucosa and sharp carinae. He had, however, complained of three small haemoptyses in the previous six months. The presumed cause, a very small tumour in situ at the orifice of the posterior basal segmental bronchus, is clearly seen. Biopsy: carcinoid adenoma.

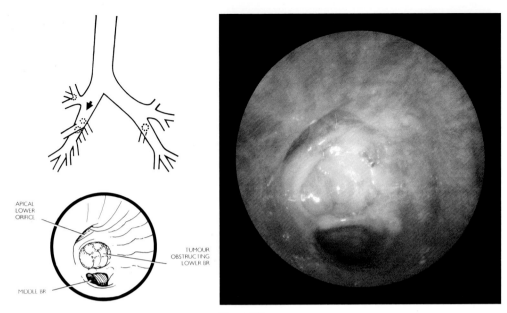

Plate 171

Hamartoma. Right apical lower bronchus. For eight months this patient had repeated chest infections accompanied by wheeze and pain in the right chest. Two years previously he had suffered a right lower lobe pneumonia. There was a persistent wheeze heard at the right base. The right apical lower bronchus has a double origin: one orifice just proximal to the middle bronchial orifice, the other (obscured) just distal. A smooth, lobulated tumour is seen obstructing the lower bronchus. This proved very hard in texture and was removed completely, in one piece via the bronchoscope, with minimal bleeding. Its origin proved to be in the more distal of the two apical lower bronchi. Histology: benign osteolipochondromatous hamartoma.

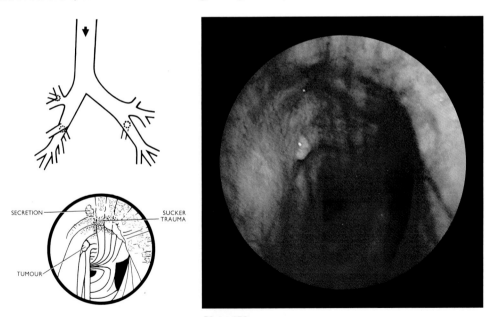

Plate 172

Papilloma. Trachea. The lower third of the trachea is visible with carina and main bronchi in the distance. The posterior mucosal corrugations are prominent and small collections of secretion are seen where they have been swept downward by the bronchoscope. There is a little traumatic bleeding on the posterior wall. Nestling on the right lateral wall is a small, rounded, yellow tumour with thin, smooth, overlying mucosa. This was removed easily and totally with one bite of the cup forceps. Such tumours are rare and easy to miss if small: this one could easily have been mistaken for a bead of secretion. Histology: benign, squamous-cell papilloma.

137

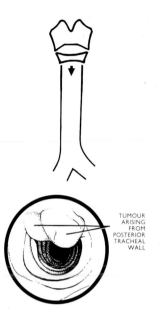

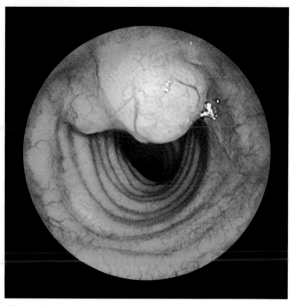

Plate 173

Lipoma. Upper trachea. Mild, generalised bronchitic changes are present. On the posterior tracheal wall lies a large, bilobed, soft and slightly mobile tumour. The overlying mucosa looks healthy. This tumour, very rare in the bronchial tree, was a fortuitous finding and had caused no symptoms. Biopsy: benign fibrolipoma. (Compare Plate 76.)

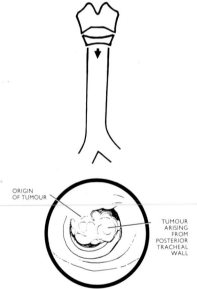

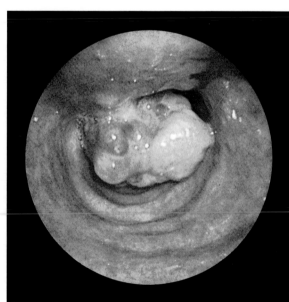

Plate 174

Metastasis from hypernephroma. Trachea. It is very rare for extrathoracic tumours to metastasise to bronchial walls and present intraluminally; they are usually deposited in the pulmonary parenchyma and are not detectable bronchoscopically. In this case, some months after removal of a kidney containing an hypernephroma, the patient complained of slight dyspnoea and a small haemoptysis. The radiograph was normal. A large, lobulated tumour is seen, with a posterior origin, one third of the way down the trachea. Biopsy: identical histology to the hypernephroma removed by nephrectomy. This tumour was successfully removed at tracheotomy. (Compare Plates 131, 133, 175 & 211.)

138

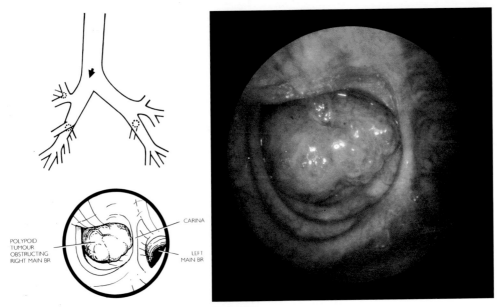

Plate 175

Metastasis from mammary carcinoma. Right main bronchus. This patient underwent mastectomy two years previously. She complained of increasing dyspnoea and wheeze for six months. A large, fleshy, lobulated, polypoid tumour arises from the posterior wall of the right main bronchus and almost fills the lumen. Biopsy: Mucoid adenocarcinoma, similar to that removed at mastectomy. (Compare Plate 174.)

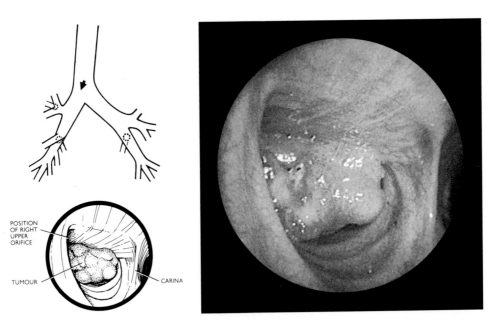

Plate 176

Chondroma. Right main bronchus. Partially occluding the right main bronchus is a large, irregular tumour arising from cartilage in the lateral bronchial wall, just beyond the upper bronchial orifice. The tumour was of hard consistency with healthy, smooth, overlying mucosa and was successfully removed by bronchotomy. Histology: simple chondroma. (Compare Plate 50.)

139

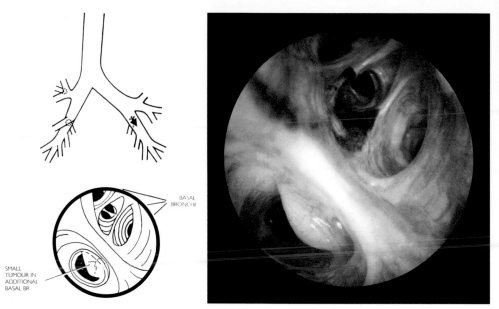

Plate 177

Multiple chondromata. This bronchitic patient was bronchoscoped following an exacerbation of symptoms and recent haemoptysis. The mucosa is diffusely inflamed with mucopurulent secretion present. Bleeding occurred readily (as can be seen here due to sucker trauma). No other cause for haemoptysis could be found. An incidental finding was multiple, scattered, sessile tumours. One is shown here in the additional left basal bronchus present in this patient. Biopsies: simple chondromata. (Compare Plates 34, 92 & 189.)

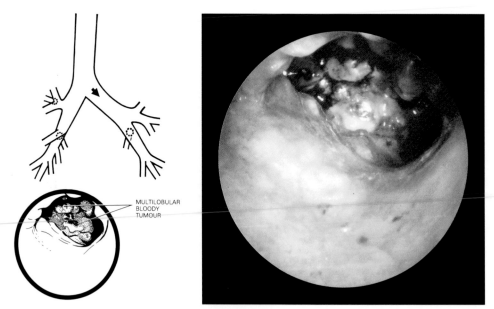

Plate 178

Oesophageal carcinoma invading left main bronchus. This patient presented with many months of weight loss and increasing difficulty with swallowing which had recently precipitated coughing and haemoptysis. Finally, he developed left lower lobe pneumonia. Oesophagoscopy and bronchoscopy were performed at the same session. There was an obvious oesophageal tumour and also a widespread, multilobular, bloody tumour erupting from the posterior wall of the left main bronchus. Both biopsies: primary oesophageal carcinoma. Subsequent necropsy confirmed direct bronchial invasion from the oesophagus with fistula at this site, clearly responsible for the aspiration pneumonia.

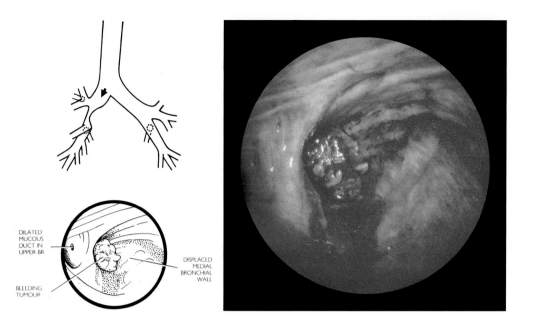

DILATED
MUCOUS
DUCT IN
UPPER BR

BLEEDING
TUMOUR

DISPLACED
MEDIAL
BRONCHIAL
WALL

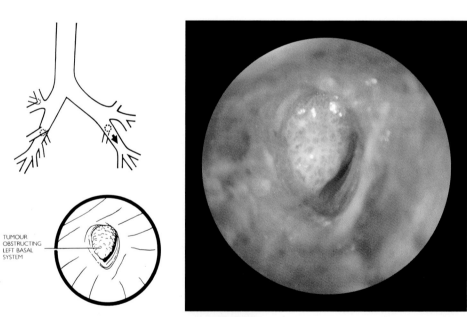

TUMOUR
OBSTRUCTING
LEFT BASAL
SYSTEM

Plates 179 & 180

Bilateral carcinomata. Right intermediate and left lower bronchi. A known bronchitic with emphysema, this patient had developed a new, persistent wheeze during the previous few months: this had disappeared recently. For six weeks he had suffered repeated haemoptyses, often profuse: he needed blood transfusion on admission. Chest radiography revealed collapse of the right lower lobe. Plate 179 shows a large, fleshy, bleeding tumour arising in the lower bronchus and almost obstructing the right intermediate bronchus: there was still an air passage to the middle lobe, for this was not deflated. The medial wall of the intermediate bronchus is displaced laterally, indicating mediastinal node involvement. The onset and subsequent cessation of a persistent wheeze is readily explained by the partial and then complete obstruction of the lower bronchus. Plate 180 shows the unusual finding of a second tumour on the contralateral side; a small, nonhaemorrhagic carcinoma arising in the left basal system. This case illustrates the importance of always examining both sides of the bronchial tree, whenever this proves feasible. Biopsies: both tumours were squamous-cell carcinomata, that on the right being less well differentiated. (Compare Plate 144.)

141

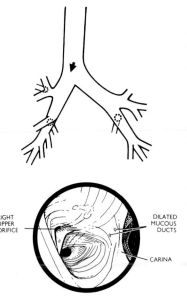

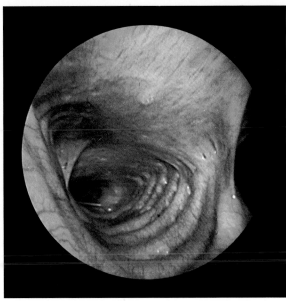

RIGHT
UPPER
ORIFICE

DILATED
MUCOUS
DUCTS

CARINA

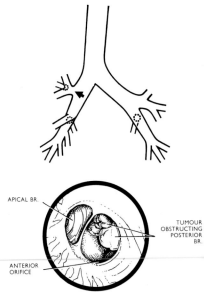

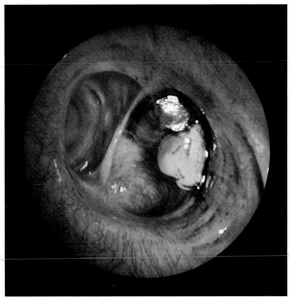

APICAL BR.

TUMOUR
OBSTRUCTING
POSTERIOR
BR.

ANTERIOR
ORIFICE

Plates 181 & 182

Carcinoma. Right upper bronchus. Importance of thorough examination. Bronchoscopy was undertaken because the radiograph revealed collapse of the posterior segment of the right upper lobe. Plate 181 shows a remarkably normal right main bronchus, apart from some senile mucosal atrophy and dilated mucous ducts just to the left of the very sharp carina and on the inferior lip of the right upper orifice (Compare Plates 58 & 130.) This lip projects into the main bronchial lumen, clearly indicating the position of the upper bronchial origin: a not unusual anatomical variation. No further pathology could be suspected from this view alone. Plate 182 illustrates the importance of inspecting every orifice possible. In this case a lateral-viewing telescope has revealed a tumour obstructing and erupting from the posterior segmental branch of the upper bronchus; thus accounting for the radiographic finding. The tumour is an example of the occasional pleomorphic behaviour of bronchial carcinoma. It presents in two parts: the lower, yellow, nodular mass and the upper, smooth, blood-stained fleshy portion. Biopsy: poorly differentiated squamous-cell carcinoma.

142

CHAPTER 9

TAKING SPECIMENS

Introduction

Obtaining specimens from the bronchial tree during endoscopy is a vital part of diagnosis. Material may be procured by aspirating bronchial secretions; by bronchial lavage; by rubbing or scraping with brush or curette; and by nibbling with suitable biopsy forceps. In addition, certain materials, such as blood clot, or very tenacious or inspissated exudate, may have to be removed piecemeal with forceps if sucking fails. Specimens can also be obtained by passing instruments through the bronchial walls: for example peripheral biopsies of lung tissue or needle aspiration of subcarinal lymph nodes. Great care and gentleness are essential during all these procedures for the sake of both patient and instruments.

Materials obtained in these ways can be examined bacteriologically, cytologically, histologically, or by other special techniques, according to suspected diagnosis and suitability of the material. To increase the diagnostic yield, it is wise to take multiple specimens in various ways for subsequent examination: one method may give the answer when others do not, and it is by no means always the same one that is successful. The material obtained is treated according to the dictates of the local pathology service.

The choice of specimen-taking instrument depends on the depth of the lesion within the bronchial tree. Forceps usually are best for any visible lesion, but it is wise to take additional specimens for cytology. The brush and fine sucking tube are more useful in smaller branches where the forceps become inoperative or if no tumour tissue is visible. Under radiographic control, remarkably peripheral lesions can be sampled: but this can be a very tedious technique and many prefer percutaneous needle biopsy in such cases.

Secretions

With a specimen trap in circuit, gross specimens of secretions can be obtained directly via the aspirating channel of the fibrescope. Maximum yield is obtained by drawing a little normal saline through the instrument at the end of the operation. A more refined method, particularly useful for aspirating individual samples from selected small bronchi, is to employ a syringe attached to a very fine polythene tube that will pass through the aspirating channel. The tube, containing secretions, is

143

then cut into short lengths and sent to the laboratory in a dry specimen container. There is minimal evaporation with this method and the specimen remains remarkably fresh and undiluted.

With the rigid bronchoscope, the removal of specimens is usually simple, using a long polythene sucker tube. A trap, clipped to the side of the instrument trolley, is included to receive the specimens. If the sucker is lodged upright in a quiver* when not in use, rather than laid on the trolley, there is less danger of dislodging other instruments from the trolley during the frequent use of the sucker; an altogether more orderly routine is possible. After each use a small quantity of normal saline is passed through the sucker by the instrument nurse to draw all removed material into the trap and ensure patency for immediate further use.

The utmost gentleness is necessary when removing secretions: they frequently obscure a lesion which will bleed freely and easily, occasionally even dangerously, if subjected to suction (Plates 185 and 186). Even careful handling of the bronchofibrescope, rigid tube or separate sucker, can produce minor trauma and this must be recognised to avoid diagnostic confusion (Plates 33, 92, 177 & 189): all chances of a clear diagnostic view may be irretrievably lost by a careless aspirating technique. Such bleeding can be greatly minimised by advancing extremely cautiously under direct vision while also listening for the first sound of successful sucking: the aspirating tube or fibrescope is then immediately withdrawn a short distance and the field inspected before proceeding further. Advancing cautiously, step by step, will be far more rewarding, both in diagnostic success and in saving time, than trying to remove secretions rapidly and completely in one movement (Plates 183 and 184).

When using rigid apparatus, it is advantageous to remove the secretion around a lesion under telescopic vision, so obtaining conditions very similar to those enjoyed during fibreoscopy. This can usually be accomplished quite easily by passing the plastic sucker tube and forward-viewing telescope together down the bronchoscope sheath (Fig. 19). This is the author's routine practice.

The behaviour of secretions or tissues on gentle sucking can often be of great diagnostic value. It may sometimes, for instance, be difficult to determine at first sight whether one is observing purulent material only, or a necrotic growth with associated infection. Gentle use of the sucker may rapidly resolve any doubts (Plates 187 and 188).

Brushings

Brushings taken from the surface of areas suggesting tumour tissue frequently give positive diagnoses. The method is particularly useful in small bronchi, where the forceps will not open, or when used blindly where a tumour beyond vision is suspected.

The brush is most conveniently introduced via the fibrescope. It is usual to employ a fine polythene tube which can be passed down the operating channel with the brush *in situ*. When the tip of the fine tube reaches the area to be sampled, the brush is protruded, rubbed on the suspicious tissue, or plunged a number of times into the suspected bronchus, and returned to the tube. This can then be withdrawn

*A 55 cm length of 2.5 cm diameter metal or plastic tubing is convenient and adequate for this purpose.

without losing sampled material in the fibrescope channel. If the brush is of the disposable type, its head, still in a short length of tubing, can be cut off and sent to the laboratory for immediate processing. Alternatively, smears may be prepared directly in the operating room by spreading the material onto glass slides and immersing in fixative.

Brushes are much more flexible than biopsy forceps and it may be possible to sample a visible, distal lesion that cannot be reached with the forceps.

Endobronchial biopsy

The most critical bronchoscopic manoeuvre is taking the biopsy: this should always be performed under telescopic vision. The bronchofibrescope fulfils this condition; the specimen obtained is very small but usually adequate because its source can be clearly chosen. When using a rigid tube, an instrument combining forceps and telescope is most suitable, so duplicating the provisions of the fibrescope (Fig. 20). If one can see clearly what the forceps jaws are gripping, it is obviously safer than a semiblind procedure: too large or inappropriate a bite into tissue to be sampled can lead to torrential haemorrhage from a pulmonary vessel or the tumour itself (Plates 193 and 194). Furthermore, it is much easier to

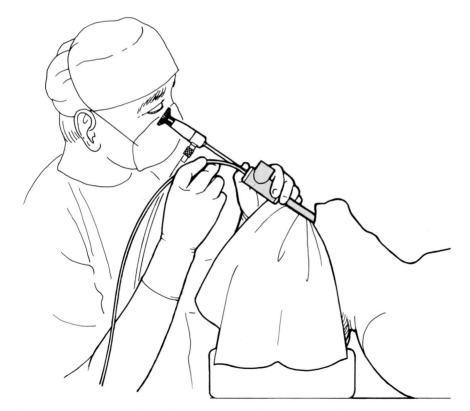

Fig. 19 Removing secretions under rigid telescopic vision. The forward-viewing telescope is held in place by the operator's left thumb while the sucker tube is manipulated under telescopic control. This technique is more accurate and less traumatic than nontelescopic operating. It is essential if the cleanest possible blood-free field is required for photography.

obtain the precise piece of tissue required under these more controlled conditions (Plate 190).

Well-adjusted cup forceps must be used so that it is not necessary to tear or pull tissue to obtain a specimen. Pathological material will usually come away easily and very gentle, small bites will rapidly give information to delicate fingers, allowing a safe biopsy to be completed (Plates 191 and 192). Large specimens are not necessary for diagnosis provided they are taken from the right place (Plate 190). All specimens so obtained are placed in 10% formol-saline for transport to the laboratory.

When using the fibrescope, the forceps should only be inserted through the operating channel when the tip is in the neutral, forward-viewing position, i.e., withdrawn to at least a main or lower bronchus; insertion through the already flexed tip of certain instruments may cause mechanical damage. If any sucking has already been necessary, irrigating the channel or possibly complete withdrawal for cleansing, will be needed before inserting the forceps, to avoid extrusion of aspirated material into the field of view. During the processs of withdrawal it will, of course be necessary to memorise accurately the location of the lesion to be sampled. During return to the lesion, the forceps should just be visible in the field of view. This ensures that the jaws are outside the flexible portion of the fibrescope; attempts at flexing without this precaution can also damage the control mechanism. It should be appreciated that the presence of the forceps reduces the flexibility of the fibrescope; thus, it is not always possible to reach the previously visible lesion for biopsy.

In the case of the rigid bronchoscope, the tube is eased into the most advantageous position possible by carefully adjusting the patient's head position, the depth to which the tube is passed, and the placement of its distal orifice. The lesion should be close to the bronchoscope tip and well within the visual field. The operator's left hand must now be so adjusted that he holds the tube firmly but gently in position, leaving the right entirely free for operating.

Reaching the lesion will now be easy in the majority of cases. The rigid operating forceps, with integral telescope, will be held differently according to the exact location of the area to be biopsied (Fig. 20). For taking a specimen from the right of the field of vision it will usually be found best to have the telescope to the left, leaving the forceps on the right, nearest the lesion: the instrument is turned through 180° for the reverse situation. Individual conditions vary considerably, however, and a trial of different positions is desirable.

A cherry-red tumour, suggesting great vascularity (for example carcinoid), or one that bleeds readily on touching, should not be biopsied, particularly when using the fibrescope without a rigid tube in place: copious haemorrhage can easily be produced. A successful technique that may be used in these circumstances, when biopsy is essential to determine future management, is to arrange for a small dose of radiotherapy to the tumour: this reduces its vascularity and allows safe biopsy a week or two later (Plates 197, 213 & 214).

Certain tumours present to the bronchoscopist much more proximally than their point of origin. It is important to appreciate this at bronchoscopy, and to establish the point of origin if possible, for the patient may prove much more treatable than appears likely at first sight, or, at least, have symptoms relieved. Gentle nibbling

146

away of the tumour to the limit of feasibility may be attempted: tumours vary considerably in vascularity and great care is necessary, but such an operation is often possible. This is, of course, a much more practical proposition with the larger forceps available at rigid bronchoscopy. A good example is shown in Plates 195 and 196: although arising from the apical lower bronchus on the left, the tumour had obstructed the main bronchus and risen, in peduncular fashion, to carinal level before driving the patient to seek advice. Removal of the intraluminal portion piecemeal allowed prompt re-expansion of the lung and also accurate localisation of the main tumour for subsequent radiotherapy. (See also Plates 160 & 165; compare Plate 159.)

There will often be cases where a lesion can be seen, but not reached with the forceps. In such cases biopsies can be taken from an area as close to the lesion as possible: a small biopsy, including mucosa and submucosa, may often reveal cancerous infiltration proximal to the main growth. In such cases, suckings and brushings obtained for cytology may be diagnostic when biopsies fail.

Finally, it is important to ensure that all bleeding has stopped before removing the bronchoscope and that any blood that may have entered the contralateral

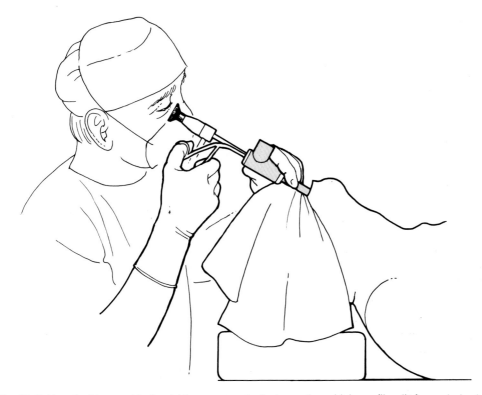

Fig. 20 Taking the biopsy with the rigid apparatus. An instrument combining a fibre-lit forward-viewing telescope and cup forceps is being used. The bronchoscope tube is held firmly in relation to the patient's upper jaw by the left hand hold described in Chapter 4. The right hand manipulates the forceps and telescope in relation to the bronchial lesion and to each other; this takes some practice to perfect but becomes automatic with experience. In this case, the forceps lies towards the operator's right, the telescope towards his left. This allows the forceps jaws to bite most easily into the carcinoma tissue found on the lateral wall of the right main bronchus.

147

bronchial tree is carefully removed, so minimising the risk of bronchial obstruction and infection.

Needle aspiration

Sometimes the best chance of reaching a diagnosis bronchoscopically, when no intraluminal lesion is found, is to obtain biopsies from enlarged lymph nodes that are obviously distorting bronchi. Transbronchial needle aspiration is the safest technique here, through either the rigid or flexible bronchoscope, particularly if confined to the widened carina (Plate 106). The author uses a wide-bore needle, sufficiently long to project beyond the bronchoscope tube, to the side of which is attached a channel for the forward-viewing, rigid, fibre-lit telescope. This allows accurate puncture of the node under telescopic vision. A small ball is soldered to the needle, 1.25 cm from its tip, to prevent too deep an insertion. Strong aspiration with a syringe will remove tissue which can subsequently be expelled from the needle for cytological examination. Suitable needles are also available commercially for the fibrescope.

Transbronchial lung biopsy

Bronchoscopy also provides one of the safest ways of obtaining *small* biopsies of the lung parenchyma. The procedure can be helpful in elucidating diffuse diseases which have defied diagnosis by other means. It is sufficiently safe and nontraumatic to be used in sick patients in an effort to discover a treatable cause for pulmonary shadowing: for example possible *pneumocystis carinii* infection in immunosuppressed patients.

Nevertheless, the fullest of possible precautions should be taken to avoid haemorrhage and reduce the risk should this occur. Blood urea, platelet count and clotting factors should all be normal and the blood group known and serum saved. Some authorities recommend instillation of 10 ml of 1/50 000 adrenalin solution into the peripheral area to be biopsied and also a prior endobronchial biopsy to reveal unsuspected poor haemostasis.

The tip of the fibrescope is wedged in the chosen bronchus. Long, flexible cup forceps are then introduced, via the operating channel, and gently passed towards the periphery of the lung until the closed jaws wedge in a small peripheral bronchus. The forceps are then withdrawn 1 cm. During inspiration the jaws are opened again and then advanced during expiration. Pulmonary tissue will usually enter the jaws and can be removed by closing and withdrawing the forceps at the end of this phase. If pain is produced (due to biting into pleura) the jaws should be opened and the procedure repeated in a new location. It is normally possible to determine whether the biopsy has been successful because lung expands and floats, whereas bronchial tissue does not.

The possible complications of this procedure are pneumothorax and haemorrhage. Pneumothorax occurs in about 10–15% of cases and, therefore, samples should only be taken from one lung. It usually presents no problem, but may need simple aspiration of the air or intrapleural drainage with suction for 24–48 hours. It can be minimised by avoiding the right middle lobe, where it is easy to pass the forceps through the oblique fissure. Whether radiological control, to avoid taking biopsies near the lung periphery, reduces the pneumothorax rate is unclear and experienced operators often dispense with radiology. Significant bleeding is uncommon and the method of haemostasis depends on the bronchoscopic technique used (see 'Control of haemorrhage', below). The right lower lobe is the safest place from which to obtain biopsies: not only is the oblique fissure avoided, but the basal bronchi are the most directly accessible to the forceps, both for the biopsy itself and for subsequent control of haemorrhage, if this should become necessary.

The fibrescope alone, introduced without a rigid bronchoscope tube, is widely used for this operation, but there is seriously increased risk should haemorrhage occur. One can attempt to control bleeding by keeping the bronchus plugged with the fibrescope itself. However, blood clot will certainly adhere to the objective lens and occlude the aspirating channel so that if bleeding continues one is faced with a rapidly deteriorating situation, made worse by loss of both vision and sucking facilities. In such circumstances the presence of a rigid straight tube has the great advantage of providing a channel for drainage, large bore suckers, balloons, packing and adequate ventilation. (See 'Control of haemorrhage', below.)

The only disadvantage of the rigid tube is the loss of pleural pain appreciation during general anaesthesia.

Biopsy of peripheral lesions

Although hardly a technique for the beginner, one should mention an advance made possible by the bronchofibrescope and the delicate miniature instruments developed with it; the transbronchial sampling of peripheral pulmonary lesions. The procedure is undertaken in the radiographic department with full resuscitative facilities available. A formal bronchoscopic examination is made to exclude other obvious lesions. The fibrescope is passed into the anatomical segment presumed to be involved, as determined by previous postero-anterior and lateral radiographs, and the lesion approached as near as possible visually. From this point, further manipulation is controlled radiologically. This is achieved by fluoroscopic guidance in two planes, first of the fibrescope tip as far as it will go, and then, still more peripherally, of the forceps or brush, towards the lesion itself where appropriate specimens are taken. This sounds much easier than it is; finding the correct, often very small, peripheral bronchus can be frustrating and time consuming. It is the author's opinion that radiologically controlled, percutaneous needle biopsy of small peripheral lesions is quicker and more accurate.

Bronchoalveolar lavage

This technique allows the collection of fluid and cells from peripheral lung tissue. Cell counts and estimates of various proteins in these specimens may help in differential diagnosis of diffuse pulmonary lesions. *Pneumocystis carinii* infections may also be diagnosed by finding the organism in the returned fluid. Sterile, buffered, normal saline, usually 150–200 ml in 50 ml aliquots, is instilled through the fibre-scope, wedged in a basal bronchus, and is then aspirated by gentle suction. The procedure is usually safe, but can spread infection in bronchitics and occasionally produces hypoxaemia in ill-chosen patients.

Control of haemorrhage

Haemorrhage, following manipulation within the bronchial tree, is usually due to taking biopsies (Plate 194), but occasionally follows sucking only. If slight or moderate, continued aspiration alone, with the sucker or fibrescope slightly with-drawn from the bleeding lesion, may be all that is required while awaiting the natu-ral clotting process. If a rigid tube is in place the application of a small swab soaked in 1/1000 adrenalin solution will be the only additional manoeuvre necessary in a proportion of cases. The swab is applied to the bleeding point with gentle pressure for two to three minutes and then carefully removed. Another application may occasionally be necessary.

Profuse haemorrhage, such that blood flows in a steady stream, or is clearly of arterial origin, should be very rare if manoeuvres are always carried out with great caution and gentleness, and large cup forceps are avoided when using rigid appara-tus. However, the slight risk always exists, even when sucking, and, if the operator has no plan of action and is unnerved by what can be a truly terrifying and rapidly worsening situation, the patient's life is immediately in jeopardy. Blood may rapidly fill the bronchial tree and pour from the mouth or rigid bronchoscope. Vision is immediately obscured and, unless appropriate action is quickly taken, the bronchial tree will fill with blood, causing asphyxia. This will be followed by cardiac arrest and death. Without following certain cardinal rules there will be little hope of controlling the situation: these are set out below.

A. Bronchofibrescope

The difficulty of controlling continuous bleeding following biopsy via the fibre-scope has already been referred to in Chapter 3 and earlier in this chapter. Although rare, the risk of death is real and the incidence due to uncontrolled haemorrhage during pernasal bronchoscopy is reported as between 0.01% and 0.1%: the higher figures are associated with transbronchial lung biopsy and thus, for this procedure, it is very important to take the preoperative precautions pre-viously mentioned on page 148. Advice relating to the control of haemorrhage with a bronchofibrescope is set out numerically below.

1. Wherever possible, before taking the bite, (especially during transbronchial biopsy) *the tip of the bronchoscope should be wedged in the appropriate segmen-tal or subsegmental bronchial lumen*: at this stage the instillation of 10 ml of 1/50 000 adrenalin is advised by some.
2. If significant bleeding does occur after the biopsy (as must be assumed if vision is obscured by blood in spite of suction) *the wedged position is maintained for at least five minutes* to allow a clot to form.
3. The fibrescope can now be partially withdrawn and will probably bring at least part of the clot with it.

4. An attempt is made to clean the bronchofibrescope lens on the mucosa and, if unsuccessful, to clear the suction channel with saline. A final precautionary inspection and bronchial toilet can be carried out if bleeding has stopped.

5. It may be necessary to withdraw the bronchoscope completely for adequate cleansing before this can be achieved.

6. *Great care must be taken not to disturb any residual clot near the source of bleeding.*

7. It most cases no further action will be necessary: continued suction for a few minutes will usually deal with any slight continued bleeding.

8. With some fibrescopes, the above 'plugging' technique cannot be applied in the upper lobes because the forceps will not negotiate a sharply curved operating channel: the specimen can only be obtained by withdrawing the fibrescope, together with the forceps and biopsy in situ, to a position where it can be straightened. Furthermore it is obvious that aspiration cannot be performed until the forceps are withdrawn from the fibrescope. (Here is an added reason for restricting lung biopsy to the basal segmental bronchi wherever possible.)

9. Haemorrhage following biopsy of a proximal tumour may cause even more serious problems because the above method cannot be applied in this situation: the usual fibrescopes cannot be used to obstruct a bronchus of greater diameter than approximately 5.0 mm. However, it may be possible to keep pace with the bleeding and maintain an adequate view of a proximal biopsy site by continuous aspiration: this may be necessary for many minutes. The instillation of adrenaline solution (10 ml of 1/50 000) can be useful.

10. *If bleeding exceeds suction capability, thus obscuring vision and removing any certainty that the patient is not drowning, the supine, head-down position must be adopted.*

11. It may still be possible to obstruct the appropriate bronchus *by introducing a No. 4 Fogarty balloon catheter through the operating channel, provided one is sure that the fibrescope tip is still appropriately placed.*

12. If bleeding continues at this stage *there is no alternative to attempting the insertion of a rigid bronchoscopic tube and then proceeding as described under B below.* There are three major problems here. First, the majority of operators today have no experience of rigid bronchoscopy. Second, unless in extremis, or under general anaesthesia, the patient is conscious and will resist the attempt. Third, vision for intubation may be totally obscured by blood pouring up the trachea and filling the pharynx and mouth. The only advice that can be given here is to *attempt the insertion with a large bore sucker tube already in the bronchoscope sheath and presenting at the leading end.* Sufficient blood, hopefully, can then be continuously removed to allow vision at the critical point during the insertion attempt.

B. *Rigid bronchoscope*

1. The bronchoscope tube, the orifice of which should have been as near the point of biopsy as possible before taking the bite, *must not be moved until the bleeding has stopped. The firm left hand grip on sheath and upper jaw must be maintained to*

prevent movement. Following the sheath to its tip with the sucker will be the only way of finding the bleeding point once vision has been lost: *moving the sheath may lead to a completely irretrievable situation.*

2. *The operating table must be tilted head down,* so that blood runs out of, rather than into, the bronchial tree.

3. *Strong suction must be applied, with a wide bore aspirating tube,* to keep the field as clear as possible: an accurately placed adrenalin-soaked swab may still prove adequate if the bleeding point can be located accurately.

4. If this proves ineffective, *pressure must be applied to the bleeding point.* This can be done by using a balloon occlusion catheter* or by packing the bronchus with a suitably sized gauze swab introduced with grasping or biopsy forceps. This is then left in place for at least five minutes plus any additional time necessary for the patient's clinical condition to stabilise.

5. While the bronchoscopist is dealing with the haemorrhage the anaesthetist, or other assistant, should *start an intravenous infusion,* arrange cross-matching and send for transfusion blood if control is not rapidly obtained. Plasma may be needed while awaiting the blood. The advantages of having the intravenous line already established for the anaesthetic, and oxygen Venturi ventilation in operation, will be obvious in this emergency situation. Such ventilation is the only truly effective method in these circumstances for it allows the operator independence of the anaesthetist.

6. When the patient's condition is satisfactory, the occlusion catheter or pack can be very cautiously and gently removed, but with another ready to hand in case bleeding recommences.

7. In many cases the haemorrhage will not recommence after removing the pack or catheter. A period of observation, and possibly further bronchial toilet, including the contralateral side, will be all that is needed. Great care should be taken at this stage not to redisturb the site of haemorrhage by incautious use of the sucker. The bronchoscope should not be removed until it is clear that the bleeding has stopped, the patient is fit, the bronchial tree is clean and at least a further five minutes have passed.

8. If further packing proves necessary, consideration must be given to thoracotomy. If the operator is not himself a thoracic surgeon, the pack or catheter must be kept in place while advice is sought.

It will be clear from this brief outline that a successful outcome not only depends on calm and competent teamwork by anaesthetist and operator, who must both follow a logical plan, but also on having the necessary forceps, swabs, balloon occlusion catheter and adrenalin always ready to hand.

It also will be obvious that the technique described cannot be adequately applied when using the fibrescope alone.

Finally, with any endobronchial bleeding, during either rigid or fibreoptic bronchoscopy, it must be remembered that there is more danger from drowning than from exsanguination. *Efficient suction for some minutes, with the patient in the head-down supine position, will be the appropriate and adequate measure in the great majority of situations.*

*Fogarty, 8 to 14F.

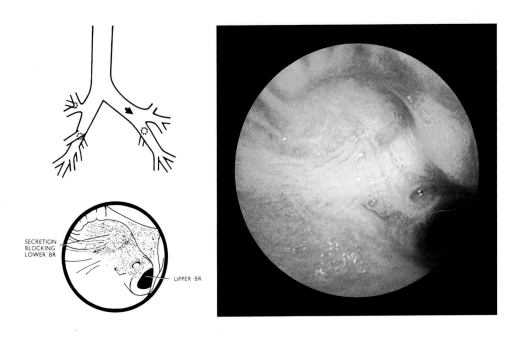

SECRETION
BLOCKING
LOWER BR

UPPER BR

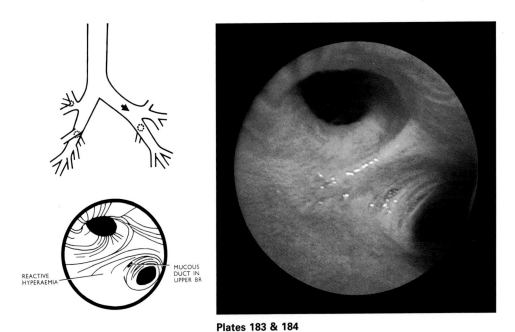

REACTIVE
HYPERAEMIA

MUCOUS
DUCT IN
UPPER BR

Plates 183 & 184

Removing secretion. Division of left main bronchus. In Plate 183, mucopurulent secretion is seen filling the left lower bronchus. It is saddling the secondary carina and is also present in the upper and main bronchi. Posterior mucosal corrugations are seen at the picture periphery, but only slight reddening is present. In Plate 184, the secretion has been carefully removed. Nevertheless, even gentle use of the sucker has produced definite reactive hyperaemia of the mucosa. The importance of gentle manipulation of instruments to avoid trauma and consequent diagnostic confusion cannot be overemphasised.

153

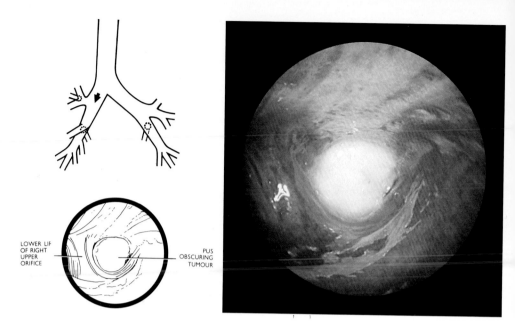

LOWER LIP OF RIGHT UPPER ORIFICE

PUS OBSCURING TUMOUR

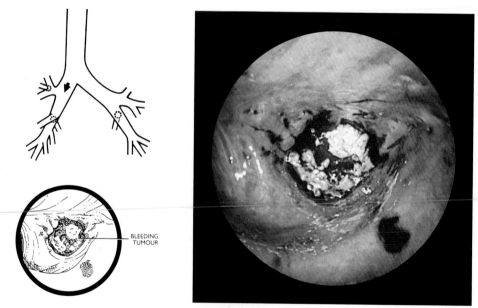

BLEEDING TUMOUR

Plates 185 & 186

Sucker trauma. Carcinoma. Right main bronchus. The carcinoma involves the lower part of the right main bronchus. In Plate 185 it is obscured by purulent secretion lying on its surface. Very careful removal of this, in the manner described in the text, can usually avoid bleeding. Unfortunately the sucker was thrust a little too deeply, so that it touched the tumour. The annoying bleeding that followed is seen in Plate 186. The photograph was taken immediately after aspirating blood and thus minimises the situation: there was, in fact, a steady oozing for some minutes. Many tumours are haemorrhagic and great care and gentleness are always worthwhile; much worse bleeding than described here can follow careless manipulations.

154

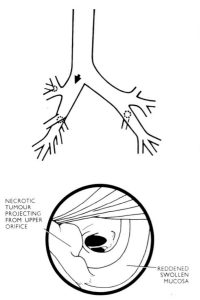

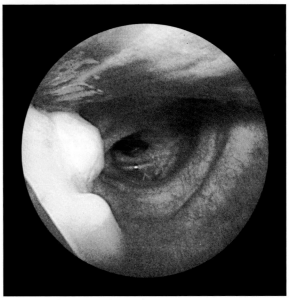

NECROTIC
TUMOUR
PROJECTING
FROM UPPER
ORIFICE

REDDENED
SWOLLEN
MUCOSA

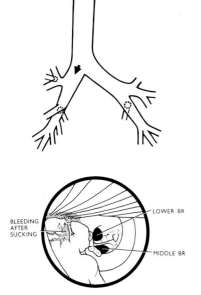

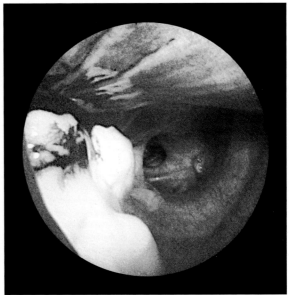

BLEEDING
AFTER
SUCKING

LOWER BR

MIDDLE BR

Plates 187 & 188

Sucker trauma. Carcinoma. Right main bronchus. In Plate 187 the carcinoma presents as a fungating, necrotic, white tumour projecting from the upper orifice into the right main bronchus. At first sight it is often impossible to determine the nature of the material seen; it could be thick, purulent secretion or tumour. Gentle use of the sucker in these circumstances can be rapidly diagnostic: Plate 188 shows that, instead of removing material as usually occurs with secretion, minor bleeding from the necrotic tumours has been produced. Biopsy was easy from this site and yielded squamous-cell carcinoma. There is reddening of the surrounding mucosa and the division into middle and lower bronchi can be seen in the distance.

155

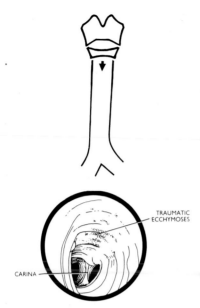

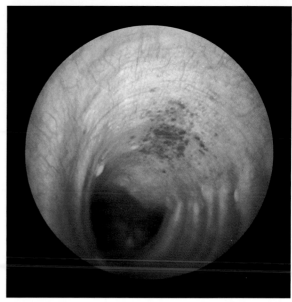

Plate 189

Sucker trauma. Trachea. There is generalised reddening of the mucosa and considerable mucopurulent secretion was present. While removing this, the sucker was allowed to touch the posterior tracheal wall: hence the multiple ecchymoses seen in the mid trachea. The damage is trivial: its importance lies in possible confusion with naturally occurring pathology. (Compare Plates 33, 92 & 177.)

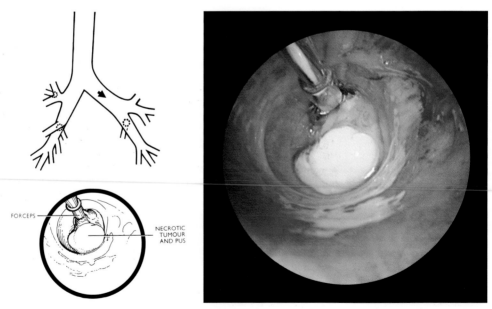

Plate 190

Taking the biopsy. The left main bronchial lumen is occluded by a large tumour photographed at the moment of biopsy. It is important that the specimen should be taken from what is likely to be a truly representative part of the tumour: here the most superficial necrotic material and pus have been avoided and the forceps jaws are seen embedded in the distal, clearly fleshy tissue. Histology: poorly differentiated squamous-cell carcinoma.

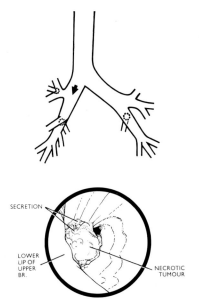

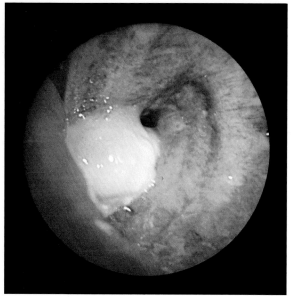

SECRETION

LOWER
LIP OF
UPPER
BR.

NECROTIC
TUMOUR

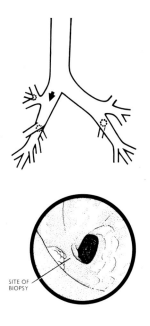

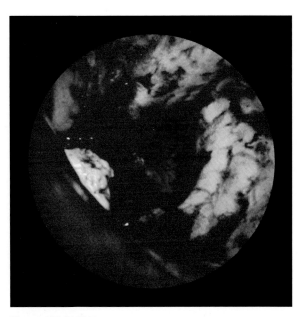

SITE OF
BIOPSY

Plates 191 & 192

Carcinoma. Right main bronchus. A large necrotic tumour partially occludes the lower part of the right main bronchus (Plate 191). Generous portions of the tumour were removed to assist in re-establishing an adequate airway, and provide material for histological diagnosis. This degree of bleeding (Plate 192) is normal and acceptable. Histology: oat-cell carcinoma.

157

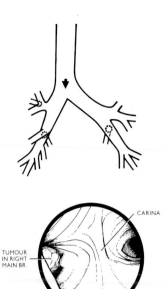

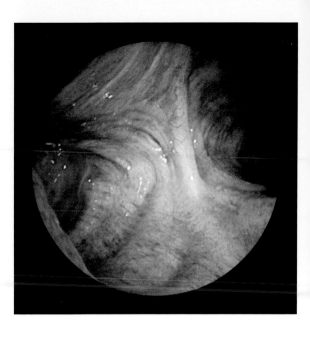

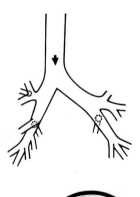

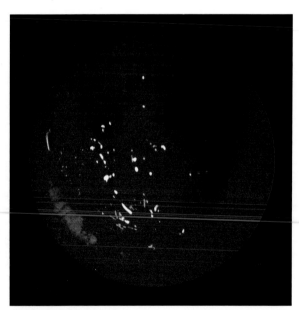

Plates 193 & 194

Haemorrhage following biopsy. Right main bronchus. Plate 193 shows a large, intraluminal tumour in the right main bronchus. There has already been a little spontaneous bleeding on its surface. Only a small biopsy was taken but copious bleeding followed. Adrenalin swabs eventually controlled this but large clots formed which, it was thought, might become dislodged and obstruct the left main bronchus. These were removed but bleeding recommenced. Eventually it was decided to leave large clots present in spite of the potential risk (Plate 194). These created no problem. Histology: squamous-cell carcinoma.

158

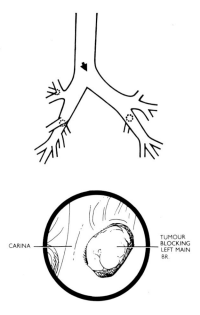

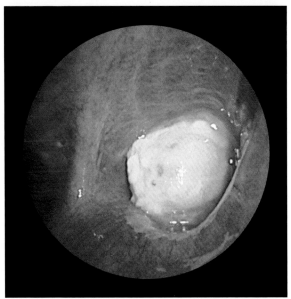

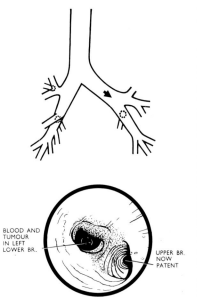

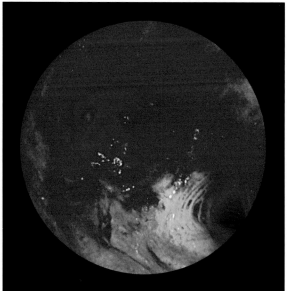

Plates 195 & 196

Bronchoscopic removal of tumour. Left main and lower bronchi. The patient presented with complete collapse of the left lung and marked dyspnoea. Plate 195 reveals the cause: a large, fleshy tumour, with necrotic surface, totally occluding the left main bronchus up to carinal level. It proved possible, without excessive bleeding, to remove piecemeal the entire intraluminal portion of the tumour. It was only attached at the orifice of the apical lower bronchus through which it appeared to be erupting. The situation following removal is shown in Plate 196, a photograph taken near the division of the left main bronchus. Blood clot is present in the lower bronchus, but the main and upper bronchi are patent again. Immediately following bronchoscopy the left lung re-expanded, excepting the apical lower segment which was now shown by radiography to contain the primary tumour. The patient experienced great symptomatic relief. Localisation of the primary site, only achieved by removing so much tumour, allowed more rational and localised treatment than would otherwise have been considered. Biopsy: undifferentiated carcinoma. (Compare Plates 160 & 165.)

159

CHAPTER 10

MISCELLANEOUS CONDITIONS

Since this is an introductory work, some of the less common but interesting conditions are briefly mentioned together in this final miscellany, rather than receiving chapters to themselves.

Bronchial bleeding (for control of haemorrhage see Chapter 9)

In many cases of reported (and confirmed) haemoptysis, the visible bronchial tree, even on very careful examination, will prove to be normal. At the other extreme, instances occur where so much blood is present in the bronchial passages that its origin is impossible to determine (Plate 197). Occasionally quite obvious and profuse bleeding has occurred, producing extensive clotting and consequent bronchial blockage (Plate 198). Such clots may be difficult to remove except piecemeal with grasping forceps. In other cases the cause of the bleeding may be obvious: a carcinoma (Plates 132, 154, 157 and 199), broncholithiasis (Plate 93), an extruding suture in a bronchial stump (Plates 233 & 234), or bronchiectasis (Plate 64) may be producing a typical endoscopic picture in addition to the bleeding. Often, however, even if a definite lesion is not discovered, bronchoscopy can be of very great value: the presence of a small quantity of fresh blood, accurately located, will indicate its lobar, segmental or subsegmetal, source. On the other hand, blood aspirated from one bronchus may clot in another, so that when bronchoscopy is performed this is the only lesion found. Careful examination of the site of the clot and a consideration of other clinical findings, particularly radiology, should elucidate the matter (Plate 200). Occasionally, although the cause of the bleeding is clear, bronchoscopy may be of great value in the patient's management (Plates 201 & 202).

The most careful, gentle intubation and subsequent examination is essential, in patients reporting haemoptysis, to ensure that no traumatic bleeding occurs to confuse the issue. Cleansing the bronchial tree by gentle lavage with normal saline may occasionally assist to locate the bleeding point.

Sarcoidosis

Although, in many cases, the bronchial tree is normal, sarcoidosis can produce two principal effects: bronchial distortion and mucosal changes. In the early stages there is often well-marked tracheobronchial lymph node enlargement giving cari-nal and subcarinal widening, with bronchial distortion frequently extending dis-tally to involve the medial walls of both main bronchi (Plate 203). This distortion may be the only finding and thus similar to that seen with benign tumours (com-pare Plates 39 & 105). In addition, however, the mucosa, particularly in the region of the carina and main bronchi, often shows a profusion of small, swollen vessels, arranged in a typical network pattern more definite than that seen in simple bron-chitis (Plate 204). Sometimes the disease may present as a subacute tracheobronchi-tis with a marked inflammatory reaction, but no features specific to sarcoidosis. In more long-standing cases, additional to reddened mucosa and the vessel network, slightly increased secretion may be present: typically this is distributed as numer-ous, small nodules (Plate 205). In many cases sarcoid granulomata may be seen in the mucosa. They present as small, yellowish swellings diffusely scattered round the carina and main bronchi. Varying considerably in size, they may imitate closely miliary tuberculosis, carcinomatosis or even the nodules of secretion (Plates 204 to 207: compare Plates 82 & 143). Plaques are occasionally found and, later in the disease, contractive scarring can distort and stenose the affected bronchi. Sarcoid tissue is commonly found in material from the abnormal mucosa and/or in lung obtained transbronchially: by undertaking both forms of biopsy in suspected cases, a diagnosis can be obtained in a high proportion of cases.

Radiation changes

Changes due to radiotherapy follow a common pattern: an immediate, acute inflammatory reaction; subsequent shrinkage or disappearance of the tumour and subsidence of the immediately surrounding inflammation; finally, some months later, local pallor of the mucosa over an area of contractive scarring and often marked telangiectasia surrounding or invading this area (Plates 208 to 214). In ad-dition, subsequent further tissue contraction and fibrosis may occur: the extent of this, and the consequent bronchial distortion, sometimes of marked degree, prob-ably depends more on the extent of the original cancerous infiltration than the dose of radiotherapy (Plates 132 & 208).

Foreign bodies

Foreign bodies in the bronchial passages, although not common in adults, have an importance far higher than their incidence for, unless a meticulously careful history is taken, they are frequently unsuspected. Apart from the commonly associated in-tense local inflammatory reactions, foreign bodies may lead to widespread infec-tion and destruction of bronchial and pulmonary tissue distal to their lodgement. Yet, if discovered in time, the great majority can be removed bronchoscopically to avoid such serious sequelae. Possible confusion with bronchial tumours has been mentioned in Chapter 8, but after careful removal of purulent secretion, which is usually present, meticulous examination of the underlying lesion, including gentle probing with forceps, will often lead to suspicion of foreign body lodgement. The ability to grip something hard or firm with the forceps, which then moves on gentle pulling, is confirmation of one's suspicions. Aspirated bones from food (Plate 215), nuts (Plate 216), pieces of denture broken off in accidents or when eating, or tacks held in the mouth when working, are the commonest foreign bodies found in adults in British practice. One case here illustrated is unusual in that the position of lodgement, on the posterior bronchial wall, has avoided bronchial obstruction. Pathological changes, even after six years, are thus restricted to local granulation tissue formation, leaving the foreign body clearly visible (Plates 217 & 218). Contrast medium, introduced deliberately during bronchography, is occasionally seen and may be confusing if unrecognised.

Tracheal trauma

Occasionally one is called upon to perform bronchoscopy immediately after a general anaesthetic has been given. Usually an endotracheal cuffed tube will have been used and this produces characteristic hyperaemia, and often ecchymoses, where it has been inflated just below the larynx. This is in marked contrast to the more distal normal tracheal mucosa and may cause confusion unless recognised (Plate 225). Bronchoscopic confirmation of tracheal or bronchial wall fracture occasionally may be needed, particularly after road traffic accidents. Rarely the problem of tracheal stenosis may be encountered: this usually has been an aftermath of tracheostomy (Plates 219 to 224).

The problem of stridor

Stridor may be recognised clinically as indicating upper airways obstruction which may also be diagnosed from lung function tests (for example flow-volume loops). Laryngeal and tracheal tomography will frequently give an indication of the level of the obstruction. Such cases should be most carefully examined first with the laryngoscope (if very high obstruction is suspected) and then with the rigid bronchoscope (Plates 97, 211 & 220): careless manipulation can precipitate oedema or bleeding serious enough to cause final occlusion. If the patient is critically dyspnoeic and the obstruction appears negotiable by fibrescope, this instrument can be used as a 'guide wire' to insert a flexible endotracheal tube. It is wise to have facilities for tracheostomy available in such circumstances. Palliative perendoscopic laser therapy can be considered in suitable cases.

Tracheopathia osteoplastica

This is a very rare condition of unknown etiology, characterised by widespread multiple excrescences arising from tracheal and sometimes bronchial cartilages. They may present as small rounded nodules (Plate 226) or protrude well into the trachea to suggest stalactites.

Amyloidosis

Amyloidosis occurs very rarely in the bronchial tree: the one case seen by the author is illustrated here (Plate 227). Yellow/grey sessile nodules appear on the bronchial walls and may suggest carcinomatous infiltration: they may be solitary, few or many, scattered in the lower trachea and main bronchi.

Hodgkin's disease

Hodgkin's disease often involves intrathoracic lymph nodes to cause bronchial distortions just as do other types of tumour. It can also involve the lung: usually the parenchyma, but occasionally bronchial tissues. There may be raised, yellowish plaques on the bronchial wall or the processes can be very much more destructive and be difficult to differentiate from carcinoma (Plate 228).

Coal deposits

Characteristically these present as glistening black plaques in the bronchi of coal miners (Plate 229), but may be found, in less florid form, in city dwellers. A similar picture is seen in the scars following intrabronchial discharge of tuberculous lymph nodes (Plate 92).

Adhesions

String-like adhesions are commonly formed during the healing process in bronchial stumps (Plate 128), and may also be seen following chronic inflammatory conditions. Rarely the cause is not ascertained and may be developmental (Plate 230).

Bronchial fistulae

Bronchopleural fistulae can occur, as a secondary problem, in the presence of empyema, lung abscess, rupture of an infected lung cyst, pneumothorax, trauma, or postoperatively (particularly in the presence of infection, such as after resection for bronchiectasis). They will, naturally, only be seen if the communication with the bronchial tree can be reached by the bronchoscope. This is particularly likely in cases secondary to thoracic surgery, when the fistula involves the bronchial stump (Plate 231). The distinctive feature is the occurrence of bubbles, in the secretions at the site, during respiratory movements.

Problems with bronchial stumps

Bronchopleural fistula, as a complication of pulmonary resection, has been mentioned above, but other problems occur which can be elucidated at bronchoscopy. Stitch granuloma essentially is a foreign body reaction seen in bronchial stumps and associated with extruding stitches. Small granulomata occur, which often suggest recurrence of tumour at the suture line (Plate 233: compare Plate 232). Usually the patient presents with haemoptysis and cough. Removal of the stitch and granuloma usually achieves a cure, unless further stitches are extruded. An extruding suture, although producing symptoms, may not always excite granuloma formation (Plate 234).

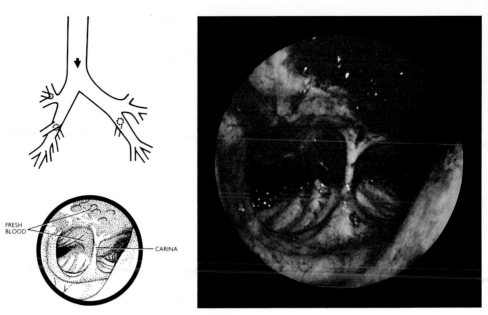

Plate 197

Profuse bleeding. Main bifurcation. This case illustrates well that accurate diagnosis is often difficult if bleeding is sufficiently profuse. All that may be achieved is a decision on the side of origin of the blood, or, more frequently, the lobar origin. This, however, may be of very considerable help in choosing appropriate therapy and bronchoscopy is always worth undertaking. In this patient blood was removed by the sucker as it welled up the right main bronchus and there was time to appreciate that it was coming from a narrowed right upper bronchus. Palliative radiotherapy to the right upper bronchus was therefore chosen and this controlled the bleeding. A second bronchoscopy, and biopsy, later established a diagnosis of oat-cell carcinoma. (Compare Plates 213 & 214.)

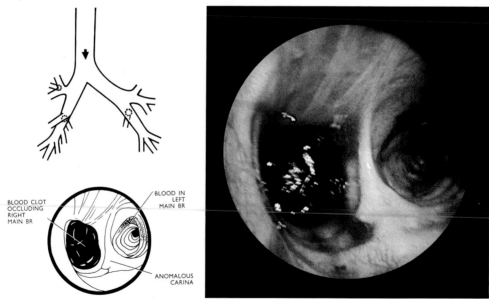

Plate 198

Idiopathic bleeding. Main bifuraction. Bronchoscopy was undertaken following one week of repeated haemoptyses. The carina is distorted by a minor developmental variation. (Compare Plates 48 and 93). The right main bronchus is totally occluded by fresh blood clot and a small quantity of blood has spilled into the left main bronchus. It needed two bronchoscopy sessions to extract all the clot, which had blocked all visible orifices on the right. The totally collapsed right lung re-expanded completely within the following week and there was no recurrence of bleeding in the following 10 years. Bronchography was normal and no cause was found for the haemorrhage.

164

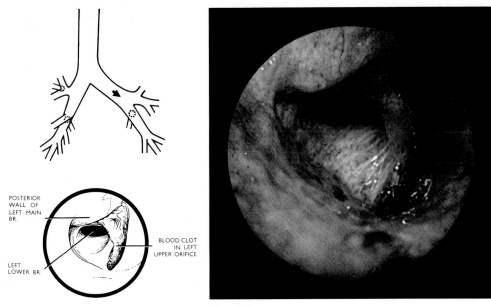

Plate 199

Bleeding. Left upper bronchus. Bronchoscopy was indicated for increased cough and minor haemoptysis in a heavily-smoking chronic bronchitic. The primary division of the left main bronchus into upper and lower bronchi is well seen. Some bronchitic changes are present. Protruding from the left upper orifice is a large, recent blood clot, with mucus on its surface. The orifice is largely occluded by the clot, but this was easily removed to reveal a vascular tumour arising within the bronchus. Biopsy: oat-cell carcinoma.

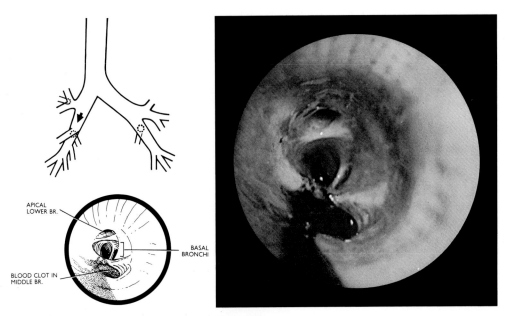

Plate 200

Blood clot. Right middle bronchus. Bronchoscopy was undertaken for minor haemoptyses and a *left* upper lobe radiographic shadow. There was no bleeding at the time of instrumentation. The findings were entirely normal, including the left upper bronchus, apart from the fresh blood clot here seen occluding the *right* middle bronchus. This was readily removed and no other abnormality was found beyond the clot. Biopsy of the middle bronchial wall revealed normal mucosa and no tumour. The diagnosis, proved by lobectomy, was adenocarcinoma in the *left* upper lobe well beyond bronchoscopic vision. Such a situation can be confusing, but subsequent follow-up for 18 months, with no further tumour developing, confirmed the conclusion that the blood in the middle bronchus had been aspirated from the left-sided tumour.

165

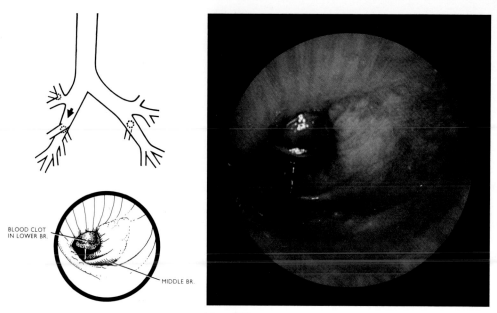

Plate 201

Organising blood clot. Right lower bronchus. An acute respiratory infection was accompanied by brisk hae-moptysis which so frightened this nervous patient that thereafter he declined to cough adequately. The right lower lobe became airless and this led to the bronchoscopy. A red-brown, smooth mass is seen partially occluding the lower bronchus. The majority of this tenacious material was removed with forceps and proved to be organising blood clot: the lobe promptly re-expanded. (Compare Plate 202.)

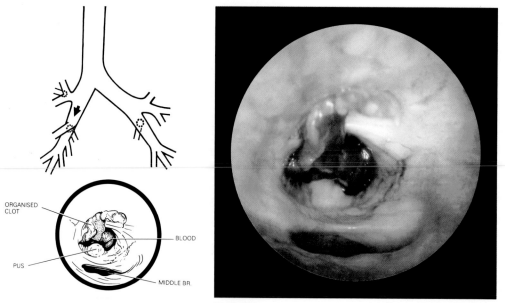

Plate 202

Organised blood clot. Right lower bronchus. This patient was admitted to hospital with a pyrexial illness associated with cough and haemoptysis. Organised yellow clot, pus and some fresh blood are seen obstructing the lower bronchus. All were removed by aspiration and no further pathology was found. The collapsed lower lobe rapidly expanded. (Compare Plate 201.)

166

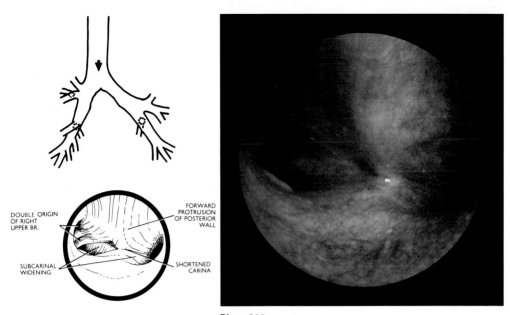

Plate 203

Sarcoidosis. Main bifurcation. This patient, with bilateral hilar lymphadenopathy, complained of dry cough following erythema nodosum one month previously. The mucosa was diffusely reddened and the dilated mucosal vessels presented as a widespread network in the lower trachea and main bronchi. This is seen here on the anterior tracheal wall in the lower part of the picture. Yellowish miliary nodules of sarcoid tissue are faintly visible. Evidence of lymph node enlargement is also striking. This has caused sufficient subcarinal widening to reduce considerably the calibre of both main bronchi. The forward protrusion of the posterior tracheal and left main bronchial walls is due to simple flaccidity and was abolished by ventilation. The right upper bronchus has a double origin. (Compare Plates 103 to 105.)

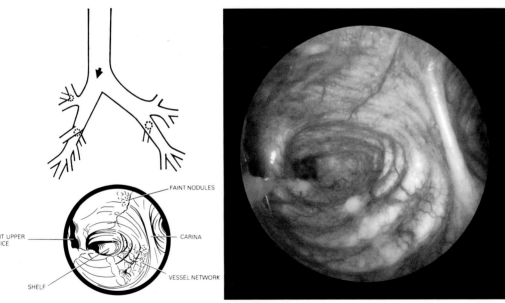

Plate 204

Sarcoidosis. Right main bronchus. This patient complained of dry cough and increasing dyspnoea for seven months. The chest radiograph was normal. The carina and upper bronchial orifice are well seen. A medial shelf and the lower bronchus are in the distance. A prominent feature is the dilated vessel network in the mucosa. This was present in the distal trachea and both main bronchi: the more peripheral bronchi were less vascular. Small nodules were widely distributed in the mucosa and can be seen faintly in this photograph. Biopsy: non-caseating granulomata containing giant cells and Schaumann bodies, typical of sarcoidosis. (Compare Plates 205 to 207.)

167

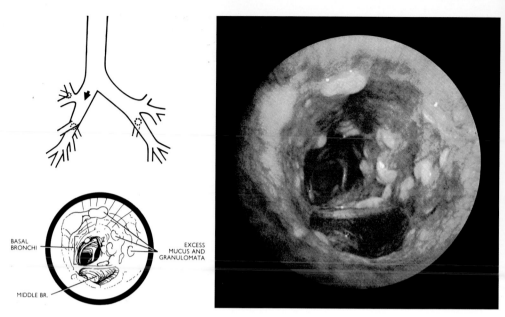

Plate 205

Sarcoidosis. Right intermediate bronchus. The patient had complained of irritating cough and minimal sputum for one year. There was bilateral mid and lower zone mottling in the chest radiograph. A normal termination into middle and lower bronchi is well seen, with generalised reddening of all bronchial walls. The most striking feature is the apparent gross, irregular, widespread nodularity of the mucosal surface. Most of this appearance is due to multiple isolated collections of tenacious mucus, which typically present in this form in sarcoidosis: a few of the nodules consist of true sarcoid granulomata. It can soon be established with the sucker which are which, and appropriate specimens obtained. Biopsy from a nodule: typical sarcoid tissue. (Compare Plates 51, 137, 138, 204, 206 & 207.)

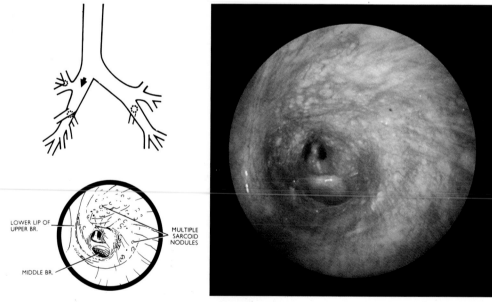

Plate 206

Sarcoidosis. Right intermediate bronchus. This patient presented with a history of dry cough for some months and bilateral hilar lymphadenopathy. Generalised mucosal reddening and swelling are evident and there is minimal displacement of the medial bronchial wall due to lymph node enlargement. The widespread granularity of the mucosa is caused by miliary nodules, here seen best on the posterior and medial bronchial walls. Biopsy: typical sarcoid granulomata. (Compare Plates 82, 143, 204, 205 & 207.)

168

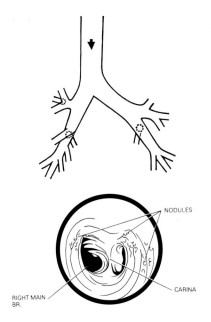

NODULES

RIGHT MAIN
BR.

CARINA

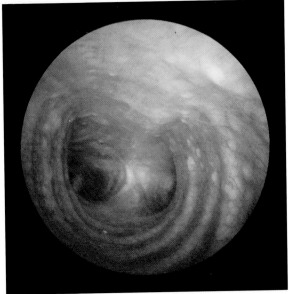

Plate 207

Sarcoidosis. Trachea. This young man complained of five months cough, malaise and aching in his joints. Chest radiography revealed bilateral hilar lymphadenopathy. There is some subcarinal widening (not clearly shown here). The mucosa shows a generalized increase in vascularity with marked reddening restricted to the trachea and main bronchi. In addition, small nodules are scattered in the mucosa over the same area. It is rather unusual to find these changes, typical of sarcoidosis, so high in the trachea. Biopsies: non-caseating granulomata typical of sarcoidosis. (Compare Plates 137, 138 & 204 to 206.)

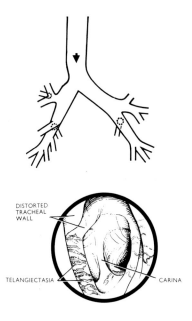

DISTORTED
TRACHEAL
WALL

TELANGIECTASIA

CARINA

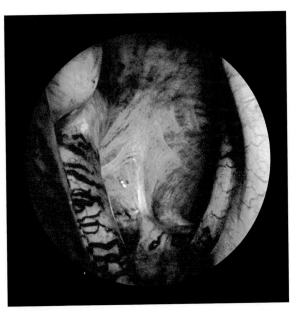

Plate 208

Radiotherapy effect. Lower trachea. The carina is well seen with a dilated mucous duct to its right. The mucosa shows generalised reddening. The right lateral wall of the trachea is the site of distortion following radiotherapy for tracheal carcinoma seven months earlier. The mucosa in this region is markedly telangiectatic; both the distortion (which can be gross) and the dilated vessels are common findings some months after irradiation.

169

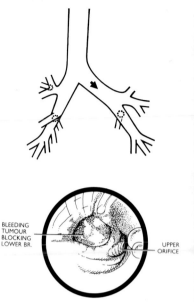

BLEEDING
TUMOUR
BLOCKING
LOWER BR.

UPPER
ORIFICE

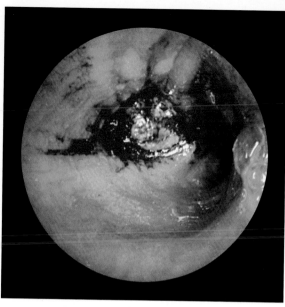

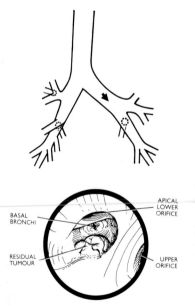

APICAL
LOWER
ORIFICE

BASAL
BRONCHI

RESIDUAL
TUMOUR

UPPER
ORIFICE

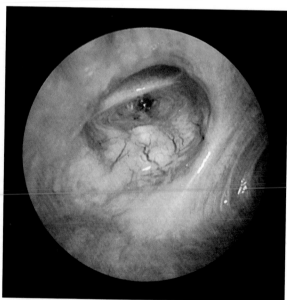

Plates 209 & 210

Radiotherapy effect on carcinoma. Cough, dyspnoea and haemoptysis were this patient's main symptoms. Plate 209 illustrates a fleshy, bleeding carcinoma completely obstructing the left lower bronchus and thus explaining the three symptoms. Biopsy: squamous-cell carcinoma. Three months later, following radiotherapy (Plate 210), a small residual nodule is all that can be seen on the anterior wall of the lower bronchus; presumably at the point of origin of the original tumour. The covering mucosa is pale, but contains prominent, tortuous vessels. A biopsy from this hard tissue, giving a tactile sensation quite unlike carcinoma, yielded fibrous tissue and no cancer cells.

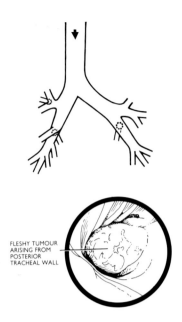

FLESHY TUMOUR
ARISING FROM
POSTERIOR
TRACHEAL WALL

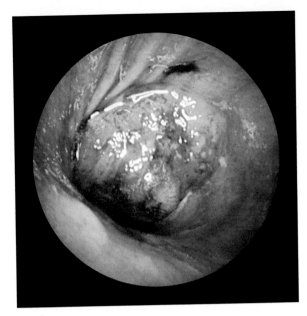

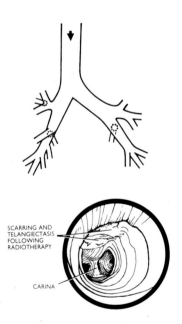

SCARRING AND
TELANGIECTASIS
FOLLOWING
RADIOTHERAPY

CARINA

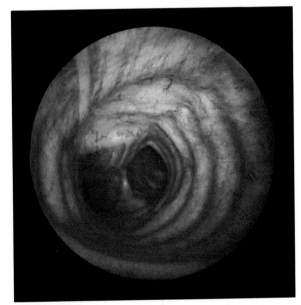

Plates 211 & 212

Radiotherapy effect on carcinoma. Trachea. Ten months previously this patient had undergone left lower lobectomy for a poorly differentiated squamous-cell carcinoma in the basal system. She now complained of repeated small haemoptyses and stridor. Plate 211, shows a large, broadly-based metastasis growing on the posterior tracheal wall and very greatly diminishing the lumen. The position three months later, after radiotherapy, is illustrated in Plate 212. The tumour has entirely disappeared to be replaced by a scar clearly delineating the original tumour base. It is typical of irradiation scars: pale, dense fibrous tissue with scattered prominent, tortuous vessels. (Compare Plate 208.) A striking feature is the destruction of the longitudinal elastic bundles: the corrugations cease abruptly at one edge of the scar and recommence at the other. This patient remained well for four years after radiotherapy and died of another unrelated carcinoma. (Compare Plates 97, 131, 132 & 174.)

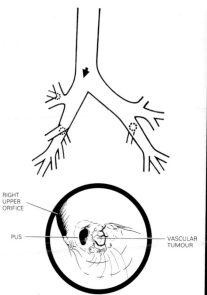

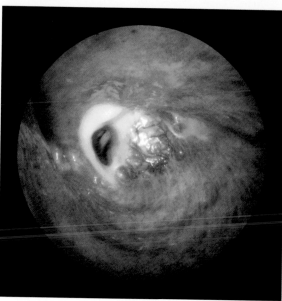

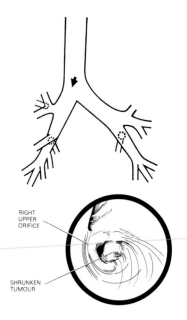

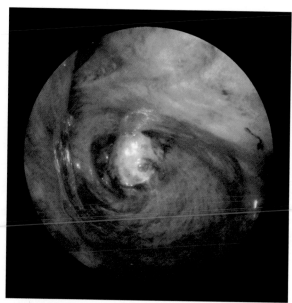

Plates 213 & 214

Radiotherapy to assist diagnosis. Carcinoid adenoma. Right intermediate bronchus. This patient had suffered repeated chest infections for some years. He reported recent, persistant, increasing cough with sputum, dyspnoea and wheeze. At the first bronchoscopy a large, red very vascular tumour was found in the right **intermediate bronchus: probably inoperable** if proved to be carcinoma (Plate 213). Removal of pus, and light touching of the tumour, led to brisk haemorrhage, raising the possibility of adenoma and successful resection. The biopsy, now considered essential for diagnosis and choice of treatment, was therefore postponed rather than abandoned. A month later, after small doses of radiotheraphy, a second bronchoscopy was performed (Plate 214). The tumour is now seen to be smaller and less vascular. Biopsy was obtained easily, without incident, and confirmed the suspected diagnosis of carcinoid adenoma. It was subsequently removed uneventfully by simple bronchial sleeve resection (Compare Plate 197).

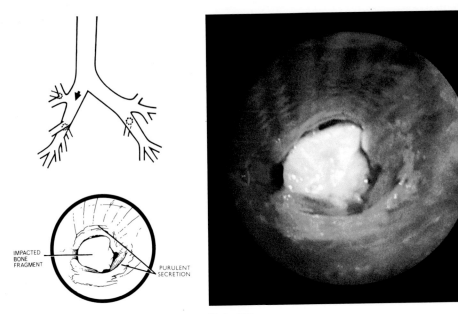

IMPACTED
BONE
FRAGMENT

PURULENT
SECRETION

Plate 215

Foreign body. Right intermediate bronchus. Obscuring pus has already been removed to reveal generalised inflammatory changes. The bronchial lumen is largely occluded by an irregular, firmly impacted, foreign body. This had been diagnosed from the history; choking over food, ensuing persistent cough and, finally, the clinical picture of right lower lobe pneumonia. Although thick pus or peduncular tumour can present similar pictures (see Plates 60, 61 & 195), whereas the foreign body has clearly retained an irregular shape. The resulting small lumina between the foreign body and the bronchial wall usually, and rapidly, become occluded by inflammatory oedema and exudate, but in this case can still be seen. The object, removed with some difficulty, proved to be the greater part of a sheep's vertebral transverse process. (Compare Plate 216.)

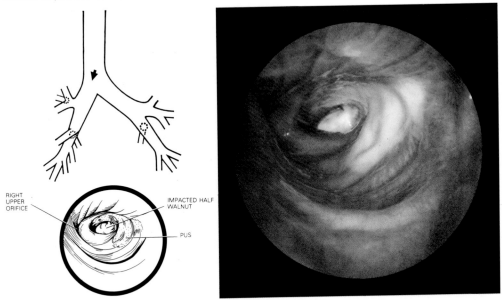

RIGHT
UPPER
ORIFICE

IMPACTED HALF
WALNUT

PUS

Plate 216

Foreign body. Right intermediate bronchus. This patient presented with a history of irritating cough and minimal sputum for some weeks followed by a febrile illness with increase in the cough and sputum. There is generalised reddening and swelling of the mucosa, with pus present. Impacted in the intermediate bronchus, coated with pus but retaining a sharp outline, is the foreign body. This was removed with ease and proved to be half a walnut. The patient's symptoms rapidly resolved. He was unable to recall any episode which could suggest inhalation of a foreign body. (Compare Plate 215).

173

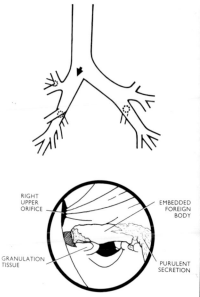

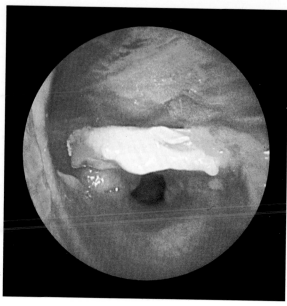

RIGHT UPPER ORIFICE

EMBEDDED FOREIGN BODY

GRANULATION TISSUE

PURULENT SECRETION

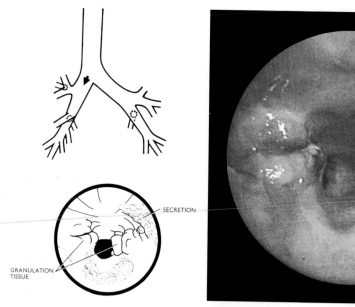

SECRETION

GRANULATION TISSUE

Plates 217 & 218

Foreign body. Right main bronchus. Plate 217 shows a flat, elongated foreign body applied to the posterior bronchial wall just beyond the upper orifice and embedded in granulation tissue. The surface is encrusted with white, dried exudate and gives the object its gleaming appearance. It was removed via the bronchoscope and proved to be a portion of denture which had been lost in an accident six years previously. Plate 218 illustrates the exuberant granulations in which it was embedded. They are the result of six years of chronic irritation and secondary infection. The inflammatory reaction subsided following the extraction and at repeat bronchoscopy six months later only firm nodules were present, with the same general outline as seen here, but with pale, healthy overlying mucosa. The patient's previous symptoms of cough, sputum and haemoptysis rapidly subsided. Immediately before bronchoscopy the chest radiograph was entirely normal.

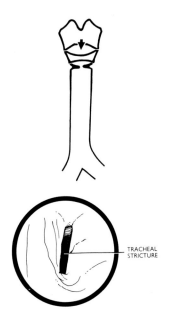

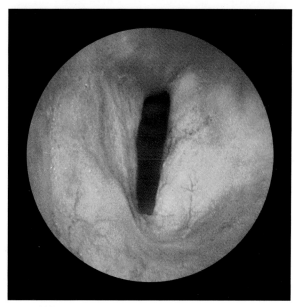

Plate 219

Tracheal stricture. The first part of the trachea, with swollen mucosa obliterating the cartilage outlines, is clearly seen narrowing to a vertical slit which proved to be slightly smaller than the glottis. Once the stricture was negotiated, the bronchial tree beyond was found to be normal. The stricture followed temporary tracheostomy performed many years previously. It gave no symptoms. (Compare Plate 220).

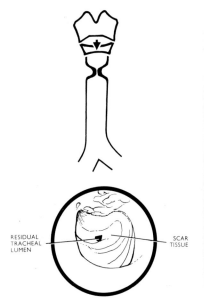

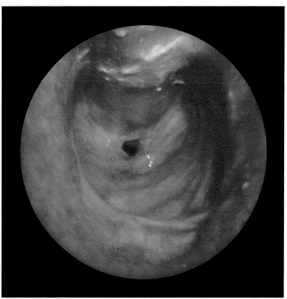

Plate 220

Tracheal stricture. The patient was admitted to hospital as a case of status asthmaticus, but the loud stridor in both inspiration and expiration, the acute dyspnoea and panic, in a patient with no previous respiratory history, and the story of a tracheostomy during treatment for tetanus six weeks previously, led to emergency bronchoscopy. The mucosa is reddened and swollen, largely obscuring the cartilages: there is some mucoid secretion lying on the posterior wall. A fibrous stricture has developed at the site of tracheostomy and reduced the tracheal lumen to about 4 mm. Urgent symptoms were relieved by dilatation. A trial of weekly bougi dilatations was undertaken, but proved unsatisfactory. Eventually surgical removal of the strictured segment of trachea was successfully undertaken. (Compare Plate 219).

175

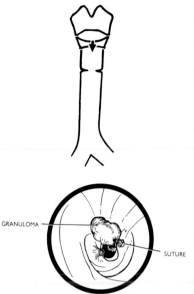

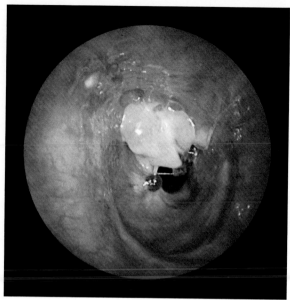

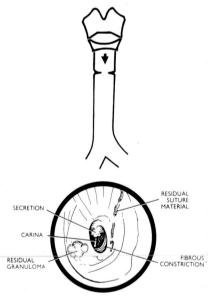

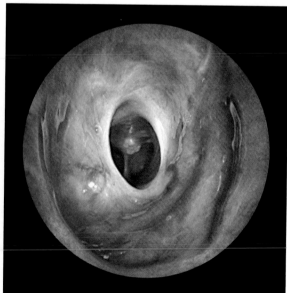

Plates 221 & 222

Tracheal surgery: stitch granuloma. This is the same patient as illustrated in Plate 220 but five and six years later: she complained of increasing stridor and irritating cough. Plate 221 clearly shows the cause. At the site of the tracheal cuff resection a pinkish-white tumour is seen arising from the posterior tracheal wall. Stitch material is embedded in its surface. Anterior to this is a small nodule on the lateral bronchial wall with a fleck of blood on its surface. Beyond this the trachea narrows, but a very adequate lumen exists. The stitch and granuloma were removed bronchoscopically and the patient's symptoms disappeared. A year later (Plate 222) there had been no recurrence of the granulomatous reaction, although suture material could be seen in the mucosa. The small nodule and moderate, residual stricture remain unchanged. Some mucoid secretion lies just proximal to the carina.

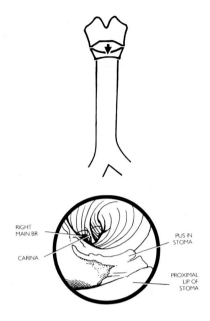

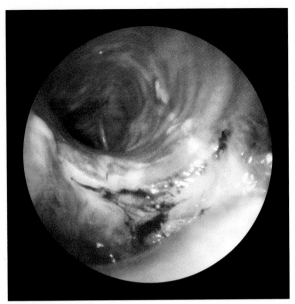

RIGHT
MAIN BR

CARINA

PUS IN
STOMA

PROXIMAL
LIP OF
STOMA

Plate 223

Tracheostomy stoma. Following a fall, resulting in a fractured femur, this emphysematous patient developed a respiratory infection with respiratory failure. Tracheostomy became necessary to maintain adequate ventilation. Bronchoscopy was performed for thorough bronchial toilet while the tracheostomy tube was being changed. Some purulent infection is seen at the stoma with generalized reddening of the tracheal mucosa.

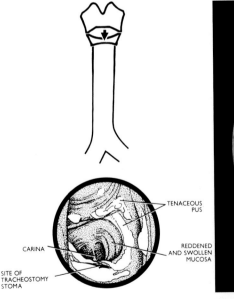

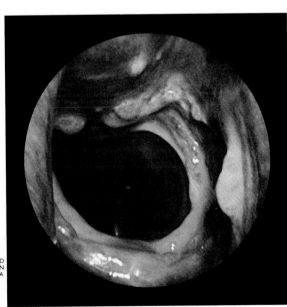

TENACEOUS
PUS

CARINA

REDDENED
AND SWOLLEN
MUCOSA

SITE OF
TRACHEOSTOMY
STOMA

Plate 224

Infection associated with tracheostomy. Tracheostomy was performed when this patient became very ill following haematemesis while in status asthmaticus. Recovery was interrupted by pulmonary infection leading to abscess formation (see Plate 61). Rigid bronchoscopy was performed following removal of the tracheostomy tube. The source of the abscess is clear; there is gross infection of the stoma and trachea, shown by swollen dusky-red mucosa and copious thick pus. Recovery was accelerated by thorough bronchial toilet and antimicrobial therapy.

177

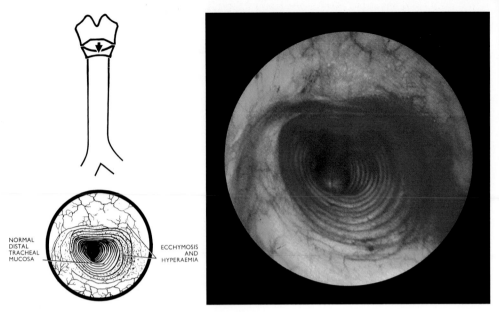

Plate 225

Reaction to endotracheal cuffed tube. Since bronchoscopy may be performed following endotracheal anaesthesia, administered for other operations, it is important to appreciate that minor, but visible, trauma is produced by the cuffed tube. Here the reactive hyperaemia and ecchymoses due to local trauma are clearly seen just beyond the larynx and contrast with the normal tracheal mucosa seen in the distance. (Compare Plate 33).

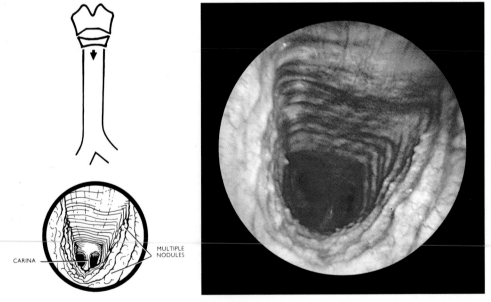

Plate 226

Tracheopathia osteoplastica. Trachea. This was an incidental finding in a heavily-smoking, bronchitic patient bronchoscoped following recent lower lobe pneumonia suspected of being secondary to bronchial carcinoma. This was confirmed. The posterior tracheal wall shows chronic inflammatory changes, but the main pathology consists of multiple, very hard, nodular excrescences, with normal overlying mucosa, on all the tracheal cartilages. Biopsy: tracheopathia osteoplastica.

178

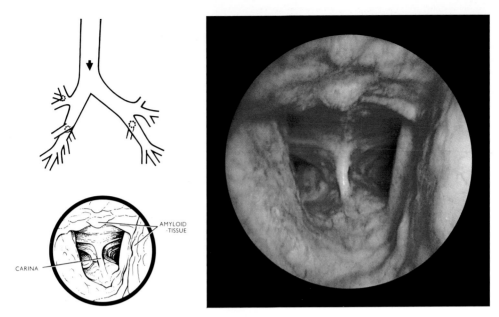

Plate 227

Amyloidosis. Lower trachea and carina. The mucosa is generally reddened but is also made irregular by numerous small, sessile 'tumours'. At bronchoscopy these were thought to be carcinomatous in origin but biopsies revealed amyloid tissue. No cause for this was found at the time, but six months later the patient was rebronchoscoped following an haemoptysis. This time an additional squamous-cell carcinoma was found in the left main bronchus.

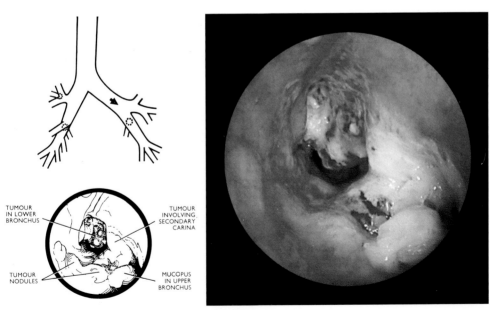

Plate 228

Hodgkin's disease. Division of left main bronchus. There are diffuse inflammatory changes in the mucosa. The upper bronchus is largely occluded by mucopus. The secondary carina, between upper and lower bronchi, is grossly widened and distorted by tumour. Nodules of tumour have appeared in the bronchial wall to give the irregularity seen on the left of the picture. A large destructive mass lies on the posterior wall of the lower bronchus. Cartilage came away easily with the biopsy specimen from this area: this revealed tissue diagnostic of Hodgkin's disease.

179

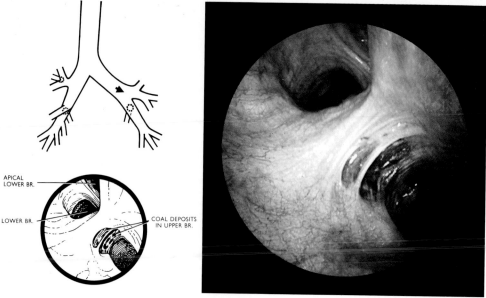

Plate 229

Coal deposits. Division of left main bronchus. The postero-lateral location of the apical lower orifice, although less common on the left than on the right, is well within normal variation. The mucosa shows gener-alised reddening and increased vascularity, compatible with this coal miner's long history of cigarette smoking. Bronchoscopy was performed following minor haemoptyses. Widespread mucosal coal deposits were an incidental finding, here particularly well seen in the left upper bronchus. The increased mucosal vascularity was considered the most probable cause of the haemoptysis. (Compare Plate 92.)

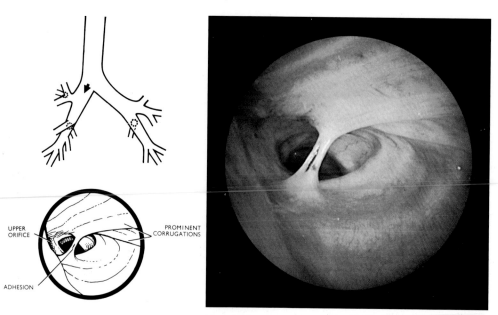

Plate 230

Adhesion. Right main bronchus. The mucosa appears healthy but the longitudinal corrugations are prominent and there was an increase in mucoid secretion. The small flecks of blood have followed use of the sucker. Opposite the upper orifice, a twin-stringed adhesion bridges the main bronchial lumen, passing from a corrugation on the posterior wall to a broad base on the anterior wall. This was a chance finding: whether congential in nature, or due to inflammatory reaction is not known. (Compare Plate 128).

180

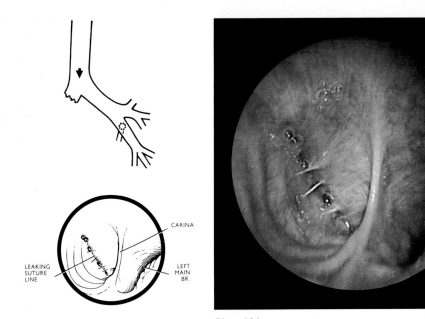

Plate 231

Bronchopleural fistula complicating right pneumonectomy. Carina and main bronchi. This patient had a right pneumonectomy for extensive bronchiectasis. He did well at first, but subsequently the fluid in the right chest became purulent. The bronchial stump is seen here; the suture line is gaping slightly and, between the sutures, bubbles are reforming after careful removal of secretion. This confirms the diagnosis of bronchopleural fistula. The patient's subsequent progress was a tragic downhill course.

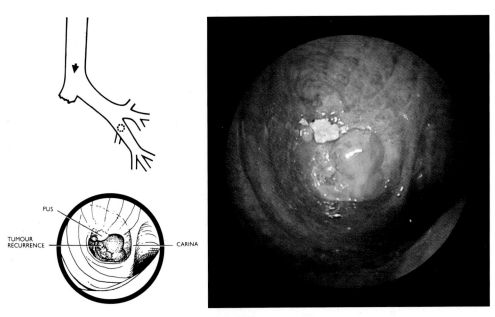

Plate 232

Recurrence of carcinoma in pneumonectomy stump. Main bifurcation. Right pneumonectomy had been performed nine years previously for squamous-cell carcinoma. Recently the patient had developed persistent cough with minimal sputum. Apart from some reddening of the mucosa the carina and left main bronchus appear normal. The right main bronchial stump is grossly involved in a fleshy, lobular tumour mass. There is a small satelite nodule on the right bronchial wall. Some purulent material lies in its vicinity. Biopsy of tumour: identical histology to that found in the right lung. (Compare Plate 233).

181

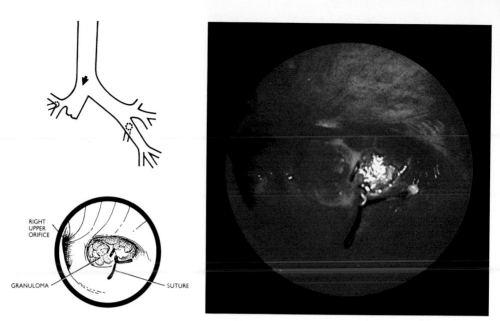

Plate 233

Stitch granuloma. Right main bronchus. This patient had a right middle and lower lobectomy for a carcinoid tumour (the same patient as depicted in Plate 169). All went well for some months but the patient then complained of haemoptysis. This photograph reveals the cause: a stitch, partially extruded from the suture line and surrounded by tissue imitating a recurrence of tumour. Stitch and 'tumour' were easily removed. Histology: granulomatous reaction to foreign material. (Compare Plates 65, 232 & 234).

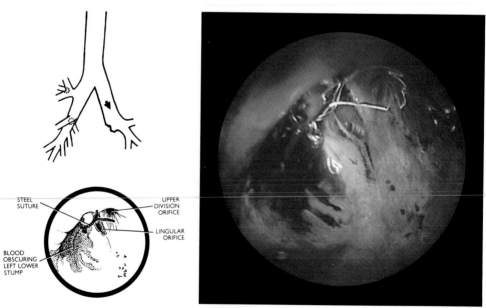

Plate 234

Bleeding from bronchial stump. Bifurcation of left main bronchus. A left lower lobectomy had been performed 20 years previously for bronchiectasis following inhalation of a peanut. A recent history of cough and haemoptysis brought the patient to bronchoscopy. Removal of the lower lobe has allowed the upper bronchus to swing downwards, so clearly revealing its bifurcation to the forward-viewing telescope. The lower stump is obscured by blood, but the steel stitch, embedded in it, is clearly visible. Bronchoscopic removal relieved the patient's symptoms. (Compare Plates 65 & 233.)

INDEX TO COLOUR PLATES

(Plates are referred to by number)

183